Moves

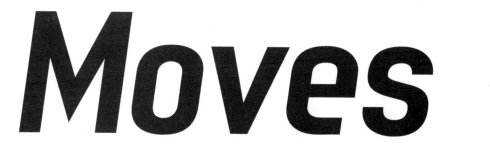

THE 4 MOTIONS TO TRANSFORM YOUR BODY FOR LIFE

MARCO BORGES
With a Foreword by Jay-Z

A CELEBRA BOOK

Celebra
Published by New American Library, a division of Penguin Group (USA) Inc., 375 Hudson Street, New York, New York 10014, USA • Penguin Group (Canada), 90 Eglinton Avenue East, Suite 700, Toronto, Ontario M4P 2Y3, Canada (a division of Pearson Penguin Canada Inc.) • Penguin Books Ltd., 80 Strand, London WC2R 0RL, England • Penguin Ireland, 25 St. Stephen's Green, Dublin 2, Ireland (a division of Penguin Books Ltd.) • Penguin Group (Australia), 250 Camberwell Road, Camberwell, Victoria 3124, Australia (a division of Pearson Australia Group Pty. Ltd.) • Penguin Books India Pvt. Ltd., 11 Community Centre, Panchsheel Park, New Delhi - 110 017, India • Penguin Group (NZ), 67 Apollo Drive, Rosedale, North Shore 0632, New Zealand (a division of Pearson New Zealand Ltd.) • Penguin Books (South Africa) (Pty.) Ltd., 24 Sturdee Avenue, Rosebank, Johannesburg 2196, South Africa

Penguin Books Ltd., Registered Offices:
80 Strand, London WC2R 0RL, England

Published by Celebra, an imprint of New American Library, a division of Penguin Group (USA) Inc. Previously published in a Celebra hardcover edition.

First Celebra Trade Paperback Printing, January 2010
10 9 8 7 6 5 4 3 2 1

Celebra Trade Paperback ISBN: 978-0-451-22897-0

The Library of Congress has cataloged the hardcover edition of this title as follows:

Borges, Marco
    Power moves: the four motions to transform your body for life/Marco Borges;
    with a foreword by Jay-Z.
        p. cm.
    ISBN 978-0-451-22607-5
    1. Exercise. 2. Physical fitness. 3. Nutrition. 4. Diet. I. Title.

GV481. B633 2009
613. 7—dc22   2008033693

Set in Bembo
Designed by Pauline Neuwirth

PRINTED IN THE UNITED STATES OF AMERICA

Power

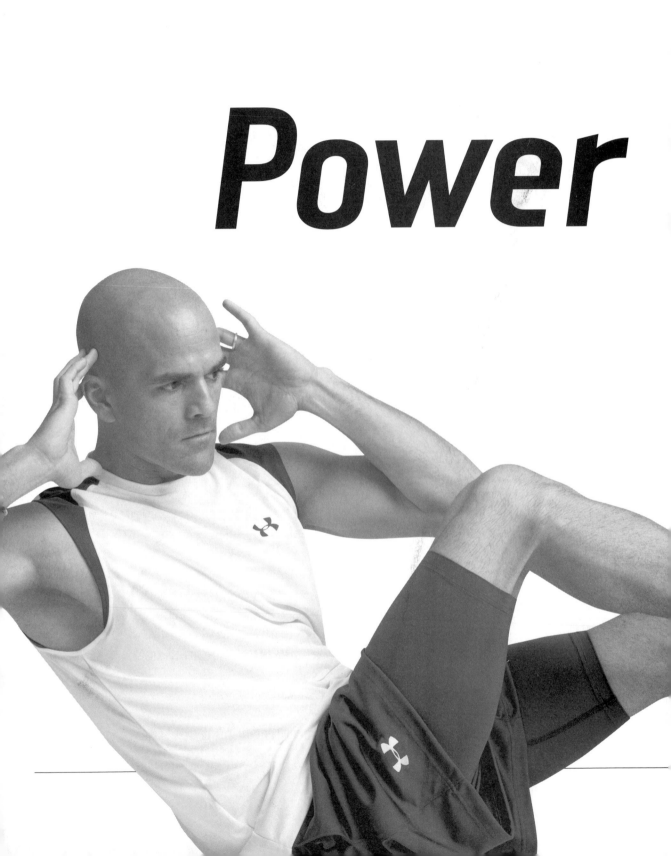

To my wife, Marilyn, and son, Marco, Jr., for their love,
support, inspiration, and so much more.
Also to my mother, Esther, my brother, Alfredo,
and my sister, Jennifer, with lots of love.

Contents

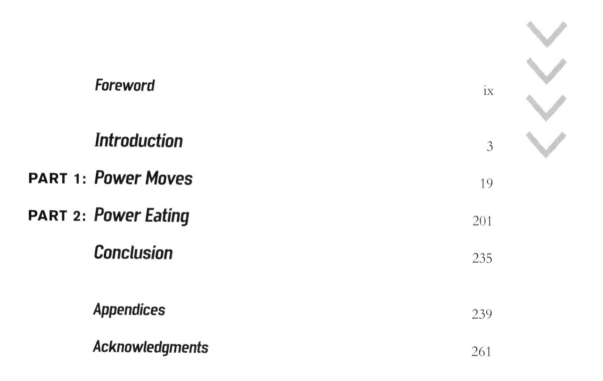

Foreword

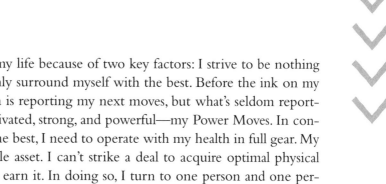

I've had success in my life because of two key factors: I strive to be nothing short of the best and I only surround myself with the best. Before the ink on my signature dries, the media is reporting my next moves, but what's seldom reported is what keeps me motivated, strong, and powerful—my Power Moves. In continuously striving to be the best, I need to operate with my health in full gear. My health is my most valuable asset. I can't strike a deal to acquire optimal physical stamina for life. I have to earn it. In doing so, I turn to one person and one person only: the world's best personal trainer, Marco Borges.

There are lots of people who are great at what they do. But then there are those who are the best of the best. It's true in all fields. What it takes to be the world's best trainer may be subjective, but to me it's all about simplicity, innovation, and motivation. Marco's approach is rooted in an incredibly simple approach: his four Power Moves. Marco focuses on moving your four major joints—shoulders, hips, elbows and knees—instead of your muscle groups. In fact, these four motions can work every muscle in your body! It sounds obvious, but once you understand how different movements of the joints stimulate different sets of muscles you can really do anything you want. Marco's Power Moves have completely redefined my notion of exercise.

I've probably gotten slightly more patient as the years have gone on, but I still can't deal with anything that's boring or just the same thing over and over. Marco is an innovator and not about routines. Every day is a new adventure. He doesn't just give you a bunch of exercises to do, or a bunch of rules about what to eat and

Marco's Power Moves have completely redefined my notion of exercise.

what not to eat. He teaches you how to *think* about your health and fitness so that you can create your own workouts, and so that you can understand how your body functions and how it is affected by the foods you eat. Ultimately, Marco has taught me that you don't need a gym or even a lot of time for that matter. You just need the will, which he motivates me to build. Once his philosophies creep into your head, you will never be the same. You will always know that the power to become the best is in you.

In this book, he gives it all up. He shows you how to make the most out of your workouts, by strengthening and toning all of the most important muscles that are stimulated when your joints are engaged, and he imparts his life-changing knowledge and practical thinking about food that will forever change how you eat.

Now don't get me wrong: I'm a "foodie." I like the best of the best, from sushi at Nobu to cheesecake at Junior's in Brooklyn. So I'm not one of these people who never eat anything that's high in fat. But *if* I'm going to eat something that's high in fat, I'm not going to waste it on junk food. I have to make it count.

The truth is, I *have* changed my eating habits over the years, and a lot of that is due to Marco. He taught me, largely by his example, to think about food in the same rational, clearheaded way that I think about everything else in my life, my business and my music—you have to earn your pleasures before you can indulge. I still eat all the things that I love. But if I know I'm going to be having a big gourmet multicourse dinner, maybe I'll make a point of eating a light nutritious breakfast and lunch and get in a good workout. That's the thing—life is about balance. Once you look at your health as a lifestyle and not a "diet," it makes all the sense in the world. Marco has taught me that health and fitness can be fun, and it's not about starving or depriving yourself. The truth is, I enjoy food more than ever because I value it more, and because I value my health even more.

Marco has traveled the world with me. Whether we're sprinting around a park in Poland or darting up forty flights of stairs in Taiwan—or whether we're arguing about whose playlist we're going to listen to while we're working out—we're always having fun. But you don't need to span the globe to have fun exercising and find the best in yourself. Everything you need is in this book. You have the world's greatest trainer motivating you, making you stronger and showing you how to create your own Power Moves. Use it and become the best!

—Jay-Z

Power Moves

Introduction

"We are all ultimately **responsible for** our own **health.**"

YOU *WILL* LOOK BETTER!
YOU *WILL* FEEL BETTER!
YOU *WILL* LOSE WEIGHT *AND*
YOU *WILL* GET IN SHAPE.

The beauty of it is that you will accomplish these goals not by driving yourself nuts spending every waking minute worrying about shedding pounds and burning calories. In fact, you will only have to think about *one* thing. One single thing—and that is your **health**. Your focus will be on achieving optimum health and maintaining it for life. You will learn how to establish a healthy lifestyle, and in doing so, you will see how everything else falls into place. Looking great and feeling great, losing weight and getting fit, all of this will happen—almost automatically—once you learn how to truly be healthy and empower yourself to take control of your body and your life.

The time is now. Every day is a new opportunity to live the healthiest life you can. Start today. Kick off your healthy new lifestyle right now. It doesn't matter how overweight you are, or how out of shape. It doesn't matter how far you think you have to go, or how overwhelming the task may seem at this point.

Think about it this way. **Your health is the one area—perhaps the only area—of your life in which you are almost completely in control of the results.** You are in the driver's seat. No one else. In other parts of our lives, such as our jobs and careers, we don't have this same degree of power and autonomy. We may work hard at our jobs and try to make smart career choices, but none of this guarantees success in the professional sphere. You can work your butt off in the office, but there are always factors that are beyond your control. Say you've been waiting for a promotion, but then you get passed over because the boss's son comes aboard and fills the position you had your eye on. Or after years of hard work and dedication you are left without a job because of corporate cutbacks. Life is not always fair. But your health is the one area where you *do* have a good amount of control. If you work at establishing and maintaining a healthy lifestyle, you are almost guaranteed to see positive results, success and health. Whatever you put in, you will get back. Whatever amount of energy you devote to the new healthy you, you'll see the same level of results in return. You can do it.

But it's up to you. Not your doctor, not your spouse, not your parents, not your siblings. We are all ultimately responsible for our own health. Understanding that the power is in you is the first step to becoming healthy. I did not always possess this understanding myself—I had to learn it just like you. Like most people, as a kid I never thought about eating healthy: I just ate what tasted good, including lots of junk food. What happened in my case was that I began to recognize patterns. When I ate better, I felt better. My understanding came about through a series of what I call **"Power Moments"**—epiphanies that come to you in an instant and stick with you for life.

There are certain points in your life when it all clicks and you truly "get it." I'm not talking about just having a theoretical understanding of what living healthy is all about. I'm talking about a feeling, a direct understanding of how everything is connected and how the kinds of foods you put into your body

. . . the power is in you . . .

affect your moods and overall happiness. When I was younger, I experienced three of these epiphanies, these Power Moments. At a certain point, I made a conscious decision to be the healthiest person I could be—and I never looked back.

As I grew more and more aware of how my body worked and how exercise and fitness contributed to my health, I began to realize that most of our muscles can be stimulated with four simple motions. The gist of it is that there are universal movements in exercise, movements made possible by four joints in the human body: our shoulders, elbows, hips, and knees. Ultimately, I came to believe that it is more effective and efficient to combine two or more of these movements—within the same exercise—for a total-body workout than to isolate different muscle groups (the push/pull approach, etc.).

As a trainer, I saw in my clients the reality that people have a limited amount of time and they are determined to get the most out of their workouts. I also saw how people spend a lot of time at the gym just wandering and wondering. Even the regulars at the gym often come across equipment they are not familiar with, and end up wasting time feeling puzzled.

I also noticed, early in my career as a trainer, that sometimes my clients wouldn't put forth as much energy when they trained by themselves as they did with me—and I realized it was because they were concentrating too much on the details of each exercise and not the bigger picture, the motions involved. I knew I had to streamline my approach. And so the way I achieved this was by coming up with the four movements. With these four simple motions, you can work out all the important muscles in your body. Whether you are exercising for ten minutes or sixty minutes, you are getting a full-body workout each and every time.

This was the genesis of the Power Moves program. Once my clients absorbed this fundamental approach to exercising, they would use it as a building block for their own creative workouts. They didn't need me telling them exactly what to do. Not only that, but they were seeing remarkable results—permanent weight loss and fitness for life.

And what has worked for my clients has worked for me as well. Time is a big deal for me too. As an athlete, I want the most out of my workouts. I don't want to have to spend the whole day exercising, and I don't want to have to feel guilty if I miss a day. Similarly, as a business owner, I have had to learn the art of multi-tasking in order to get everything done within a given time.

So I took all of these ideas, and I created this plan to teach you how to get the most out of your workouts in the shortest amount of time—in just about any setting, and with minimal or no equipment. And the key to it all is learning the importance of the different movements of the body.

The training programs I introduce in this book are all based on four fundamental movements, which I call Power Moves. By using these four motions and activating these four joints, you'll truly get a full-body workout and build total body strength. My Power Moves programs are accessible to people of all fitness levels, from beginners to professional athletes, and they are suited to people with a wide range of objectives and motivations—but they all stem from the same source, the four Power Moves.

These four simple Power Moves make up one of the most important tools you'll need to transform your body for life and achieve maximum health. You will enjoy all of the following benefits:

- reduced body fat
- reduced risk of many diseases
- stronger muscles/increased muscular endurance
- improved mood
- improved cardiovascular efficiency
- greater strength to combat chronic disease
- greater ability to manage weight
- strengthened heart and lungs
- better sleep
- better sex life
- feeling and looking younger
- improved confidence
- lowered resting heart rate
- greater efficiency in burning calories
- improved oxygen transport through your body
- healthier bones and joints

All of that and . . . you might actually enjoy it! Feeling healthy, feeling good, looking good. It won't all happen overnight—but it's also not just about getting fit and becoming healthier, it's about permanence, staying fit and healthy for life.

It's a lot easier to keep up than to catch up. Think about it: Imagine what your kitchen sink would look like after a week of not doing the dishes, how difficult it would be to get everything cleaned up and back in place. Now imagine keeping the sink clear by cleaning a dish as soon as you're done with it. Which of the two seems easier? It's a lot like a race: If you start with the rest of the competitors and try your best to keep up with them, it's a lot easier to finish with them than if you sat back for a while and then tried to catch up. Well, the same applies to health and fitness: If you are starting from scratch you may feel as though it's an impossible task, but as you get closer to your goals it becomes easier to keep up, maintain, and keep yourself on track.

HOW TO USE *POWER MOVES*

First you have to start with the right attitude. Your mind can be your greatest motivator or detractor. Therefore you must eliminate negative thoughts like:

"I have so far to go. I don't know if I can do it."

"It's too hard to change."

"Being on a diet is boring!"

"What if I fail—just like all the other times?"

Just start fresh, and remember—it's all in your attitude. If you think you can, you will. It's much easier to stay motivated if you think above all about your health.

You're already taking your first step to a better life: You're reading this book.

And as you read further you'll find the strength to take the steps to reach the peak of your power. One by one, you'll learn why you may have chosen bad habits in your life—and how you can put an end to them. You'll learn what to eat to lose weight and be healthy, without forgoing the foods you crave. You'll learn the best exercises for any situation, from when you're traveling on business to when you only have a short amount of time and want to perform the most concentrated workout. Finally, you'll learn how to relax and enjoy your newfound health and, most important, how to put all your new Power Moves together for a great life now.

In my sixteen years of experience helping people lose weight and transform their bodies and their lives, I've found that the four motions are an extraordinary catalyst for change. Within that time I went from training friends and people I knew, to clients at an exclusive fitness center on Miami Beach's Fisher Island, to customers at my own groundbreaking gym that I opened in Miami, and eventually to professional athletes and some of the biggest names in entertainment. But throughout my journey I've noticed the same basic pattern in all the individuals I've worked

IT'S ALL IN YOUR ATTITUDE

with. What happens is that people begin to exercise, using the four motions that are the foundation of all exercises, and then they start feeling better about themselves and are driven to continue because they like the way they look and feel. The exercise, and the good feelings that result, also trigger thoughts of overall wellness. People who have gotten hooked by the four motions tend to also become more conscious of what they're eating and drinking. So it all starts out with four motions, but then it snowballs into a whole lifestyle.

That is why this book is meant to be not just an exercise book, but rather a guide to a whole lifestyle—to establishing and maintaining healthy habits, from the way you eat to the way you exercise to the way you live. It is also meant to be a fun, interactive journey. You'll find questions, exercises, and lists to help guide you on your path to becoming a better you. You'll also find helpful tips and supplemental information in my "Power Tips" (extras to help you on your journey) and "Power Thoughts" (theories for further insight) boxes, which are scattered throughout the book. Finally, toward the end of the book, I've added some of my favorite delicious and healthy low-calorie-ingredient and menu options. Combined you will have at your disposal all the tools you need to transform your body and your life.

WHY ME? WHY NOW?

A week before I started writing this book, my wife, Marilyn, gave birth to our first child, Marco, Jr. When I looked at him, I felt everything that every father has through the ages: unconditional love, joy, and an unstoppable determination to see my son, my child, lead a happy, healthy life.

But that good, healthy life I wish for him did not come all too easily for me. My own childhood was in many ways typical but in other ways unique. I grew up in a Cuban neighborhood in Miami, and so there were cultural aspects of my diet that were different from that of most Americans. For example, I ate lots of rice, beans, and plantains, which of course are staples of Cuban cuisine. But like all kids I loved just having fun, riding my bike, playing in the streets, and doing all the ordinary things that kids do. I went to school, did my homework, and (reluctantly) went to bed early every night.

Some of my friends wanted to stay inside and watch TV or play video games when they came home from school. Not me. When I left school, around two or three p.m., and the warm sunlight hit me, the last thing I wanted to do was go back indoors. I wanted to do anything as long as I was outdoors. My older brother was one of those kids who loved to play inside, but, since he was right there with me, I'd drag him outside to play, and before he knew it we were having a great time. We didn't come home until our mom came out and yelled for us to get inside for dinner. Our jeans were dirty, we had scraped knees, and we smelled like dirt—the quintessential "before" picture in a laundry-detergent ad.

So I was always active as a kid. I wanted to run around, to move, move, and move some more. Because I was naturally so active (okay, Mom, super-hyperactive), I led a pretty healthy lifestyle—even without any formal exercise.

But food was another story.

I lived with my mother, brother, and sister. It might have been because my mother didn't know any better, but there were no discussions about the importance of nutritious food. Food was just, well, food. I didn't know that breakfast could be anything but a pastry picked up at the local bakery; that lunch could come on anything but a cardboard tray; and that dinner could be complete without heaps of white rice.

When it came to food, I was pretty much unconscious. I wasn't a kid who lived to eat; I pretty much ate what was in front of me or what looked good at the moment (usually something sweet). And diet? That was just a word that appeared in my mother's magazines.

But then one day something happened that made me start to think differently about food. On our way to school we stopped at the usual bakery and I grabbed one of the plastic-wrapped chocolate pastries and gobbled it up.

But by the time I got to school, my stomach was starting to hurt. Worse, after the school morning announcements, I developed an angry rash on my arms and face. I was sent to see the nurse, who said it looked like a food allergy. "Marco, what did you eat this morning?" I told her that I just ate a pastry. No big deal.

The school called my mother to tell her to pick me up. My mom was a single parent and she worked very hard to support us; taking time off to care for me meant she'd miss work.

On the way home, as I was scratching at the rash on my arm, I started to think about it—I felt bad that my mom had to leave work, and for some reason I just knew it was the pastry that made me sick. So I decided, from that point on, not to eat pastries. In fact, I decided not to take any chances: I began to skip breakfast completely.

Then one day during P.E. (physical education), about a week into my new "break fast," while I was running around the field, I started to feel dizzy. The next thing I remember was lying on the grass looking up at the sky. I had passed out because I hadn't eaten anything; I was running on empty.

That was my first **Power Moment**. It was the moment I realized . . .

You do need to feed your body, but you don't **need** to feed it junk.

So from that realization I continued to learn and grow and change. I started to read about nutrition—in magazines, newspapers, books, whatever I could get my hands on. While everyone else in the neighborhood was at the packaged-cake and processed-food aisles of the supermarket, I'd hunt down my newly discovered nutritious choices.

I was eager to learn everything I could about what I was eating, so I began to dissect it all. When I learned that white rice, the foundation of almost every Cuban meal, wasn't nearly as nutritious as brown rice because most of the nutrients in white rice were stripped off in the milling process, I switched. Fried plantains, out—I asked my mom to bake them instead. I was never overweight as a kid; as a matter of fact, I was always on the thin side. And just the fact that a skinny kid was passing up food was odd. My grandmother would say, "Marco, you need to eat, you're way too skinny, eat!"

To everyone else I was too skinny, and to my Cuban relatives I definitely looked sickly. But to me? I felt great! So, I only ate what I knew would make me feel good. To no surprise, it was healthy foods.

It was only a short leap from eating healthy to starting to exercise.

POWER MOMENTS

My second Power Moment had to do with exercise. My neighbors were throwing out a bunch of magazines and had set them down by their apartment front door, which was next to mine. I started rummaging through the pile and I found a small book written by Joe Weider, the exercise guru behind Mr. Olympia, Ms. Olympia, and the publishing empire that includes *Shape* magazine, *Men's Fitness*, *Living Fit*, and *Fit Pregnancy*, to name a few. In those days, Weider had written a lot of books about physical fitness and how to get healthy. After I read Weider, I started to read everything I could about fitness—and I learned that exercise was more than being active and playing outside. If I performed certain exercises, simple things that I could do at home, like push-ups and sit-ups, I could keep my body strong and my energy up. So when I woke up in the morning, I started to do a couple of moves, then again when I got home from school, and after supper. Exercise became a part of my routine.

And almost immediately I began noticing changes in my body. By just adding a few small exercises to my day, my body was transforming and I was really becoming fit and healthy.

It must have shown because before I knew it, people started asking me questions. My friends would ask . . .

"Marco, what should I do if I want to lose a few pounds?"

"Why is brown rice better than white?"

"What does a push-up really do for you anyway?"

MY LIFE, MY DESTINY

That experience of discovering exercise for the first time, and of helping others discover it, led to my third **Power Moment**. I realized—I liked it! I liked when my friends and relatives would ask me questions. I liked helping people. But, it was more than that . . .

Helping people to become–and stay–healthy was my passion.

Ever since I was a little kid, I had dreamed of becoming a doctor. And this dream only grew as I got older. I had some friends who were doctors and I would constantly ask them about what it was like. On one occasion a friend who was a surgeon invited me to sit in on one of his procedures. The patient was a middle-aged man with colon cancer. The experience of watching this medical procedure was a turning point for me because it made me realize that my real interest and passion lay in *preventing* disease, before it became a problem, more so than curing or treating it after the fact.

Looking at the patient I couldn't help but wonder if there was anything the man could have done to avoid this terrible illness. I felt so sorry for him and his family, and I wondered whether things would have been different if he had eaten healthier or exercised regularly. Of course I realized that sometimes you can be stricken by disease and it doesn't matter what you do. But even so, isn't it worth doing everything in your power to try to stay healthy and keep disease at bay?

The same day that I sat in on the medical procedure I scheduled an appointment with my college counselor—and after carefully reviewing my options I switched my college major from premed to exercise physiology. I thought that if I was able to prescribe exercise it would be a great tool to help people not only become healthy but stay healthy. And that's what I am today: an exercise physiologist.

At the time I was already training friends and people I knew, but I wanted to formalize my new career direction—so I became a personal trainer for the Fitness Center at Fisher Island, a private island with a hotel and very high-end apartments only accessible by ferry, near Miami Beach, Florida. I quickly became the most requested trainer and was completely booked weeks in advance. I loved the feeling I got when my clients would approach me and tell me how much their lives had changed since they began working with me: They felt better, looked better, and their friends and family had taken notice and complimented them.

I began to recognize the power I had to help people, but as a personal trainer I was limited to helping just one person at a time—so I decided that group exercise was the way to go. I got certified to teach Boxaerobics. My classes were a hit and from there I became certified as a Spinning instructor. The response to my Spinning classes was overwhelming too and it was then that I started to realize I needed to open my own club. One small problem, it would take money—money I didn't have.

So for the next few months I worked nights helping my friend, an artist who had a company painting murals for restaurants and stores. I saved up some money and with the help of a small business loan I was eventually able to open M Cycle Gym, the first indoor cycling gym in Miami. I was flying by the seat of my pants—no money for a receptionist or any advertising, and I was teaching every single class myself!—but soon word of mouth spread and all my classes were filled and there were huge waiting lists. Local news channels were even asking to interview me about the rapid success of this new kind of fitness center. These interviewers couldn't believe that I had the energy and stamina to teach every class myself!

From there it's been a wild ride ever since. Profiles in national magazines and papers soon followed. I went on to train a number of professional athletes. I partnered with the Discovery Channel on a "Body Challenge" health initiative and with the *Miami Herald* on a fitness boot camp for underprivileged children. I created a consulting firm (Move Fitness Concepts) that now advises and designs other clubs and fitness centers, both nationally and internationally. And I went on to work with some of the most incredible people in the world, who have entrusted me with their health and friendship.

But through it all, my primary focus has been to inspire health and wellness in as many people as I can reach. To give others the tools and knowledge to lead happy, healthy, and successful lives.

This was what I was thinking when I decided I wanted to become an Exercise Physiologist rather than a doctor. It was what I was thinking when I was a kid and I would answer my friends' questions about health and fitness. And it's the same thing I think now when I look at my son. The greatest gift I can give him as a parent is a great start. I look at him and I think: *You will enjoy a happy, healthy life. You will be filled with energy, because you have learned how to lead a healthy lifestyle, how to eat foods that are nutritious and delicious, and how to exercise regularly to keep yourself fit.*

What I say to my son, I also say to you: Learn what I have learned and you too can have a happy, healthy life.

No, you won't be starting from scratch, like my son. You might have some weight to lose and some bad habits you'll have to break. But like my son, your future is wide open. It's all yours. You can start right now. Today. Make this your own Power Moment.

POWER MOVES

All of us have three things in common:

1. Whether we think we can or can't succeed in our goal of eating well and exercising well—we are right. In both cases, we are right.

This is confusing, so let me explain. The point is that attitude is everything. What makes you any different from that superfit, beautifully healthy person you admire? Attitude. The way you *think* about your health. I have yet to meet someone who put their mind and energy toward total wellness and health and did not achieve his or her goal. So if you believe you will succeed, you're right—you will.

But conversely, if you believe you're going to fail, you're also right—you *will* fail.

POWERtips >> WHEN I WAS growing up, a kid on my block asked me, "Can you skateboard?" Even though I'd never been on a skateboard before, my answer was, "Yes." Not because I was lying, but because in my mind what I heard in that question was not "Do you skateboard?" but "Are you capable of skateboarding?" And in my mind I knew that, yes, I had it in me, I could be successful in learning how to skateboard—and so I did. Well, it's the same thing with eating healthy and exercising. If you believe you can, then you can. If you believe you can't—if you think you have bad genes, or you're too far behind to catch up, and so on—then you can't. It all comes down to your attitude.

2. We can be healthier, stronger, thinner—or anything else we want to be—with only a few simple, easy lifestyle changes.

Studies show that many of the diseases that haunt us can easily be eradicated by a change in diet and activity levels:

- A study of overweight, middle-aged people at risk for type 2 diabetes found that their risk was reduced by 58 percent by making small changes in their diet and activity levels.[1]
- Despite all our advances in medical science, cardiovascular disease remains the number-one killer in America. Dr. Dean Ornish, a pioneer in the study of heart health, found that 82 percent of people who had some form of heart disease—high cholesterol or hypertension—decreased their risk in one year of practicing dietary discretion, stress management, and three hours of exercise a week.[2]

POWERtips >> I AM A firm believer that when people fail it's not because they plan to fail but rather because, most of the time, people fail to plan. By this I mean that none of us expects that we will fail to achieve our health and fitness goals. But more often than not, we do fail. Why? Because we fail to *plan*. I can't stress enough how far a little bit of planning will take you. For example, say you're going out to a cocktail party, and you know there will be lots of unhealthy foods there to tempt you. Why not eat something healthy beforehand? This way you're less likely to eat unhealthy foods at the party, and if you do end up eating them, at least you probably won't eat as much. It's much easier to maintain a healthy lifestyle if you plan ahead. Don't just wait for time to work out, plan for it. Don't just wait until you're famished to decide what you're going to eat; plan and prepare foods ahead of time so when the time comes you are ready for a healthy meal and not something quick out of a vending machine or a drive-thru window.

3. In order to put these lifestyle changes into action, we first need to understand them, to have knowledge of the how, the why, and the what.

You probably know that a bad diet and a sedentary lifestyle are harmful to your health. You've read it over and over again in books and magazines. But do you know . . .

- what specific foods make up a bad diet—or a good one? (You might be surprised by the answers!)
- how much exercise you need to stay healthy and lose weight? (It's less than you may think!)
- the best exercises for maximum results—in a short amount of time? (Most of them don't require fancy equipment or a gym!)

I became powerful through years of study, practice, experience, and training. And I stay powerful by eating healthy, living healthy, and keeping my mind and body strong—all of which should ensure the best quality of life through the years.

How can you become powerful, too? How can you find your personal power, to live a good life, right now and in the future?

The answers are all inside this book.

What you have in your hands now is the best possible tool that exists to guide you in your journey to becoming healthy, fit, and powerful. Use this book as a lifestyle manual to establish healthy habits and transform your body and your life.

May you have many Power Moments while you read *Power Moves*. May you get strong and stay strong every single day.

Starting now.

Let's begin!

Power Moves

"The only machine you really **need to know how to use** is the one you already possess, **your body.**"

In this section I give you all the basic tools you need to become healthy, toned, slim, and powerful. While there is certainly more to being healthy than just exercising, it is an *essential* component in your overall health and wellness. It is one of the fundamental building blocks in your journey to transform your body for life.

Everything you need to know about transforming your body through exercise is all right here in this section. However, I want to be clear about one thing. These training programs are not meant to be the be-all and end-all when it comes to exercise. My Power Moves are not intended to be taken as some sort of Ten Commandments of exercise.

Any effective approach to health and fitness must be flexible, not restrictive. The reason why so many exercise and diet programs fail is precisely because of their one-size-fits-all mentality. When you tell people that they have to follow your exact set of rules, or perform the exact same exercise and routines that you do, it's a recipe for disaster. What happens is that the person inevitably veers off of the prescribed regimen, and then feels like he or she has failed—and ultimately gives up.

It's like that old proverb about how if you give a man a fish you feed him for a day, but if you teach him how to fish you feed him for a lifetime. That's how I feel about heath and fitness, and that's why my approach is to teach you how to *think* about exercise and help you understand how and why certain movements will lead to positive results.

In particular, I will teach you in this section how and why it is that focusing on the basic motions made possible by our four major joint groups—our shoulders, elbows, hips, and knees—is the key to getting the body you want.

FOUR MOTIONS TO CHANGE YOUR LIFE

The human body is made up of many joints, and these joints are what make movement possible. There are wrist joints, knuckle joints, foot joints, spine joints. But the four major joint groups—our shoulders, elbows, hips, and knees—are responsible for the majority of our bodies' movements, and so it makes sense that targeting these joints is the most simple and effective way to achieve a full-body workout.

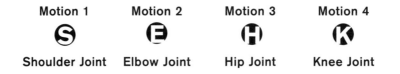

Motion 1	Motion 2	Motion 3	Motion 4
Shoulder Joint	Elbow Joint	Hip Joint	Knee Joint

These four motions hold the key to unlocking your untapped potential. By flexing, extending, adducting, abducting, and rotating these four joints, you will harness the power to build a strong, lean, and healthy body for life. Best of all, by understanding these four motions (joints), you will learn which muscles are responsible for their movement, which in turn allows you to better understand which exercises and machines target these muscles. But the only machine you really need to know how to use is the one you already possess, your body. Once you have a basic understanding of your body and the Power Moves, the function of all other machines and exercises will seem obvious.

Why are these four joints so important? Because, again, these are the places where most of our movement begins. From these four joints come flexibility and movement. From these four joints come action and function. From these four joints come strength, vigor, energy, confidence, and power.

By having you focus on these four joints—and getting you to think about the motions and the muscles involved—I'm giving you the understanding that is the foundation of transforming your body for life. The specific exercises and training programs that I introduce in this section are to get you started, and also to give you guidance based on your individual goals and motivation. But as you progress you will have the power to create your own moves if you so desire.

Now that you know the What—what the four motions (shoulder, elbow, hip, and knee) are—I will explain the Who, When, Where, and Why.

Who . . . should perform these motions? Anyone looking for a complete total-body workout.

When . . . should they be performed? A minimum of three times per week or any time you engage in resistance-training exercises.

Where . . . should they be performed? At home, the gym, a hotel, or wherever you are at the time. The beauty of these moves is that they can easily be performed with little or no equipment in just about any space.

Why . . . should they be performed? These motions are the key to engaging the major muscles of the body and achieving a full-body workout for a strong, fit, and healthy body for life.

The Power Moves workouts focus on all four motions within each individual resistance-training program, to ensure a total-body workout with whichever routine you choose.

Power Moves also focuses on many *compound exercises, which allow you to work more than one muscle group at the same time.* Some of the exercises introduced in this section are isolation exercises (move the body through only one joint movement), while others are compound exercises (move the body through more than one joint movement). A good example of the difference would be the leg extension and the barbell squat. While both target the quadriceps, the squat is a compound exercise, and in many ways it is superior to a leg extension—an isolation exercise—because the squat works so many other muscles in addition to the quads; it is really a total-body workout. This affords you shorter workout times, while stimulating maximum muscles.

Motion 1: THE SHOULDER JOINT Ⓢ

Why: Engages the muscles of the chest, shoulders, and back. Everyone wants a stronger, toned chest. But strong shoulders and back are important, too—they mean better posture, a better core, and more flexibility.

What it does: The "ball-and-socket joint" is the most mobile joint in the human body. It can abduct, adduct, rotate, and raise in many places. It has an incredible range of motion, but because of this it tends to be one of the most injured joints.

What muscles it works: Basically, the chest, shoulders, and back. More specifically, there are the *deltoids* (anterior, lateral, and posterior), which provide flexibility and a range of motion, and enable you to move your arms forward, back, up, and down; the *trapezius* muscles, which form the triangle of your shoulder and upper back; the *rhomboids*, which pull your shoulder blades inward; the *rotator cuff* (supraspinatus, infraspinatus, teres minor, and subscapularis), which enables you to move your shoulder without any pain; the *pectorals*, your chest muscles, which flex and adduct the upper arm; and, finally, the *latissimus dorsi*, which are large muscles on the outside (lateral side) of your trunk, and which extend, adduct, and internally rotate the shoulder joint.

Working it/examples: Shoulder presses, push-ups, pull-ups, dumbbell presses, shoulder flys, lat pull-downs.

Power Tips: Because of its incredible range of motion, the shoulder is often the source of pain at some point in one's life. For the most part, however, this pain can be prevented through proper maintenance of the rotator cuff muscles, which internally and externally rotate the arm (through shoulder flys and internal/external rotation). Don't neglect those little muscles and chances are you'll live with pain-free shoulders for many years to come.

Motion 2: THE ELBOW JOINT

Why: Engages the muscles of the biceps, triceps, and forearm. This joint is a great complement to the shoulder joint. The elbows are crucial in building

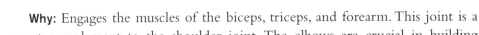

POWER THOUGHTS >>

JUST IN CASE you were in doubt, here are some recent, less-well-known studies showing how important exercise is to our health:

- Consistent moderate-to-vigorous aerobic exercise significantly reduces the risk of colon cancer in men.[1]
- It also reduces the risk of developing diabetes.
- And it also reduces the risk of premature death.
- Exercise can improve your sex life.[2]
- Regular physical activity may help reduce urinary incontinence in women.[3]
- Exercise reduces the symptoms of mood disorders.[3]
- Even low-intensity exercise, such as gentle yoga or a stroll, reduces fatigue by 65 percent.[4]
- Consistent exercise can delay biological aging by twelve years.[5]

strong, powerful, and functional arms (especially important because we use our arms in almost everything we do).

What it does: As a "hinge joint," it is involved in the flexion and extension of the humerus (upper arm) and ulna (lower arm).

What muscles it works: The *biceps* (the muscles in front of your upper arms), which flex the elbows and supinate (turn up) the forearms; the *triceps* (the muscles on the back of your upper arms), which extend the forearm at the elbow; and the *forearm* itself.

Working it/examples: Weight-bearing exercises, including biceps curls and triceps extensions, chin-ups, push-ups, and dips.

Power Tips: The arms are some of the more commonly seen muscles of the body and also a pretty good indicator of overall fitness. Keep them fit with some of our Power Moves and you'll not only look great but you'll also feel great.

Motion 3: THE HIP (H)

Why: Its primary function is to support the weight of the body (need I say more?). It is incredibly important for posture, overall strength, and power.

What it does: Classified as a ball-and-socket joint, this "synovial joint" is involved in flexion, extension, adduction, abduction, internal/external rotation, and circumduction.

What muscles it works: There are seventeen muscles involved with movement of the hip, and they are classified into four groups: adductor, gluteal, iliopsoas, and lateral rotators.

Working it/examples: Squats, pelvic tilts, pliés, lunges, skating.

Power Tips: All of the gluteus muscles run through the hip. Want a great-looking bum? Work the hips.

Motion 4: THE KNEE (K)

Why: We virtually hold up our world with our knees. It's our knees that keep us upright and stable. If you have excess pounds, your knees are what bear that extra weight—and this makes you more susceptible to injury. The knee works with the hip joints, helping to tone and strengthen the same quads and hamstring muscles as your hip.

What it does: A complex, compound variety of a synovial joint, it is involved in flexion and extension of the fibula/tibia (lower leg).

What muscles it works: *Quads, hamstrings, adductors,* and *abductors.* The knees give us the ease to walk, run, and jump with grace.

Working it/examples: Squats, leg extensions, leg curls, dead lifts.

Power Tips: The knees support virtually all of our body weight, and because of this they are very susceptible to injury. Keep them healthy by exercising them regularly and by maintaining an appropriate body weight.

POWERtips >> MUSCLES 101

Muscle is muscle and fat is fat! Ever hear someone say "your muscle will turn to fat if you stop working out"? Well, that's not true! Muscle cells will always be muscle cells and fat cells will always be fat cells. Our bodies have a fixed number of muscle cells and cannot create any more. But you can create *bigger* muscles (hypertrophy) through resistance training. In other words, the quantity of cells will remain the same, but they will increase in size. Similarly, if you discontinue exercising, you may experience some muscular atrophy (shrinking), which is the opposite of hypertrophy.

Want another great reason to watch what you eat? Fat cells are a place where your body stores energy. Your body can and will continue to create fat cells to store more energy if it needs to (if you consume more calories than your body needs). If you burn (use up) that stored energy, you are decreasing the size of the fat cells—but once your body has created them, they're there to stay. Food for thought, no pun intended.

CARDIO POWER

We've been talking about the muscles of our body, keeping them strong and toned. But we haven't yet addressed the most important muscle of all: our heart.

Importance of cardio: Why do we need cardio? Well, for starters, it strengthens the lungs, as well as the most important muscle in the body (the heart). Heart disease is the leading cause of premature death for both men and women. For this reason alone, you can see that cardiovascular fitness is very important and should never be overlooked. But if this isn't enough to convince you, you should also know that cardio exercise burns calories and reduces body fat.

I recommend that cardiovascular training be performed at least three times a week for a minimum of thirty minutes, at a heart rate of between 60 and 85 percent of your max.

Different kinds of cardio: There are many different ways you can perform cardiovascular training—running, walking, hiking, bicycling, rowing, jumping rope, swimming, skating, elliptical machines, cross-country skiing, and so on—so naturally people often ask me which is best. Above all, it's important that you choose something you enjoy, because you will more than likely remain consistent if you are enjoying yourself. I highly recommend walking. Walking is a universal aerobic exercise. It is the most popular exercise with the highest adherence/compliance rate of any other form of cardiovascular exercise. Anyone can do it, at any age, at any fitness level. And all it takes is a pair of sneakers and you're ready to go. But whichever form of cardio you enjoy the most, just remember not to overdo it. Try cross training (different forms of cardio exercise) to avoid developing overuse injuries.

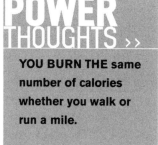

But don't be afraid to mix it up and also to do interval cardio work (where you do different forms during one workout session). Whichever form of cardio you choose, you'll be getting a lot of great benefits: stress reduction, burning extra calories, strengthening your heart and lungs, reducing the risk of certain diseases (including depression), increasing confidence and energy, and improving sleep.

Walk, run, bike, or hike, but get your cardio in. You can even use Power Move workouts to get your cardio. How? By combining your Power Moves resistance-training exercises with bursts of cardiovascular activity. In between your Power Move reps, jump rope, march in place for five minutes, or run—whatever will keep your heart pumping—then go on to the next exercise. You can also do each exercise at a faster pace. (I don't recommend combining the two until you have become familiar with the Power Move workouts.)

Benefits of combining resistance training and cardio:
Resistance training and cardiovascular training complement each other in many ways . . .

Benefits of cardio . . .
- Cardio has a high caloric expenditure, so it's great for helping you shed excess weight.

- Cardio lowers your resting heart rate, which improves cardiac function.
- Cardio strengthens your heart and lungs.
- Cardio reduces the risk of cardiovascular disease.
- Cardio helps to improve one's self-image.

Benefits of resistance training . . .
- Resistance training increases your metabolic rate, which means you will burn more calories throughout the day.
- Resistance training increases and restores bone density.
- Resistance training increases lean-muscle mass, strength, endurance, and power—so you can live better.
- Resistance training improves balance, flexibility, and stability.

And much more.

But whether you combine your resistance training with your cardio in one session, or do one or the other on different days, you will get the *benefits of both:*

- reducing the risk of cardiovascular disease
- burning calories and avoiding "middle-aged spread"
- keeping metabolism rate elevated
- increasing and restoring bone density
- improving balance, flexibility, and stability
- strengthening your heart and lungs
- building up muscle mass, endurance, and power
- lowering stress levels
- improving confidence
- increasing energy
- getting a good night's sleep

Sounds like a win-win to me!

To summarize, getting our heart rate up and sustaining it for thirty minutes not only helps our heart pump efficiently, it also helps keep our lungs strong. And, yes, cardiovascular exercise also burns calories and reduces body fat.

Okay, this makes sense. So why don't we do it? Cardiovascular disease is still the number-one cause of premature death in the world—despite everything we know, despite all our advances in science and medicine. And all it would take to lower these grim statistics is for people to take up a healthier diet, a calmer, smoke-free lifestyle, and to perform some cardiovascular exercise at least three times a week.

But how does one start? Any cardiovascular activity is better than nothing, so long as you're performing it at an intensity that works your heart.

I recommend my clients work out aerobically at least three times a week. I ask them to pick something they like to do, whether it be dancing or kickboxing or running. Or, if they argue, "I don't enjoy any kind of exercise," I tell them to pick something they dislike least! It's the same as with a job—some people really love what they do for a living, but most people aren't fortunate enough to be able to say that. So they choose, maybe not something they *love* but at least something they can tolerate, because they know they have to in order to survive.

So you should do something that you like to do, or at least something that you don't hate. But whatever cardiovascular activity you choose to do, you still have to work at it. You have to push yourself. In order for aerobic exercise to have any effect, you have to perform at an intensity that works your heart (but without injury).

Intensity: The effects of cardiovascular exercise are usually related to intensity. Intensity levels are measured as a percentage of maximum heart rate. One of the easiest and most common ways to calculate max HR is by subtracting your age from 220 (that is, beats per minute). Most cardiovascular exercise is between 60 and 85 percent of maximum HR. Begin by working out at 60 percent of that number and building up to 85 percent. For example, if you are forty years old, your maximum heart rate is around 180 heartbeats per minute. Sixty percent of that 180 is 108. Seventy percent is 126. Eighty-five percent is 153. You can either use a calculator, a heart-rate calculator online (the American Heart Association has a good chart you can follow; go to www.americanheart.org), or invest in a heart-rate monitor that "reads" your heartbeats and displays it on a watchlike face. How do you know you're working out at a pace that will give you a good workout? Use either your heart-rate monitor, or take your pulse for twenty seconds, and multiply that number by three—you should be at least at 60 percent of your HR max (maximum heart rate).

POWER MOVE WORKOUTS

Now that we've gone over the importance of cardio, we will turn our attention to the various strength-training Power Moves programs that I've created. We will cover the following . . .

1. The "No-Excuses" Workout
2. The "No-Excuses" Resistance-Band Workout
3. The "Maintain/Stay-in-the-Game" Workout Option #1
4. The "Maintain/Stay-in-the-Game" Workout Option #2
5. The "Maintain/Stay-in-the-Game" Workout Option #3
6. The "Warrior" Workout Option #1
7. The "Warrior" Workout Option #2
8. Try This!
9. Power Stretching

You're probably wondering what I mean by "No-Excuses," "Maintain/Stay-in-the-Game," and "Warrior." Let me explain. In my years as a trainer, I've noticed that the people I've come across tend to fall into three different groups.

The first group of people is made up of those who never seem to be able to find the time to work out, or those who don't enjoy working out, and so they find excuses to avoid it.

The second group is made up of those who don't mind working out or maybe even enjoy it, but their aim is just to make sure that they retain the results they've achieved.

And the third group is made up of those who strive not just to retain the results they've already achieved but to build on them to become the fittest, healthiest, and strongest they can be.

Based on these experiences with these three different groups (some people fall into all groups at different times), I've created three classes of Power Moves workouts, each designed to use those four joints—the shoulders, elbows, hips, and knees—and to work all the muscles of your body, for maximum toning, maximum fat burning, maximum looks, and maximum power!

A Few Things to Remember

Stay hydrated! Water is the most essential ingredient for life. Water has many important functions, including: the elimination of waste, transportation of nutrients, and temperature regulation. The longer and more intensely you exercise, the more important the right hydration becomes. Drink sixteen to twenty ounces of fluids two to three hours before exercise and an additional ten ounces immediately prior to exercise. Drink eight ounces every fifteen minutes of exercise and an additional sixteen to twenty ounces immediately after. Don't wait until you're thirsty to hydrate, since thirst is a sign that you are already dehydrated. Dehydration can lead to cramps, heatstroke, and even death.

Don't forget to breathe! There is limited research on the proper way to breathe when you're doing exercise, but I'm sure we can all agree—you must breathe. Here are my recommendations. During resistance training you should exhale on the exertion (difficult part) and inhale on the recovery (easy part). This is most natural and helps develop a rhythm and consistency. During cardio the most important thing is to avoid shallow breathing. Try to find a rhythm of deep breathing and try to stick to it.

Warm up your muscles. Before you begin your workout, you should walk or run in place, or use one of your gym's cardio machines for up to fifteen minutes until you've worked up a sweat.

The repetitions in each move are suggestions only. Do as little or as much as you can without feeling discomfort.

If you're not sure where to start, begin with No-Excuses. Then, move to Maintain/Stay-in-the-Game. And then to the Warrior workout. These programs are loosely correlated with different skill levels, but you can always just **increase the intensity of all three workouts by adding more weight and/or more repetitions.** The point I want to stress is that everyone is capable of ultimately performing all three workouts.

Also, you can try going faster once you are familiar with the moves of the workout you've been doing. This will add aerobic intensity to your bodybuilding.

But remember, these workouts don't take the place of cardio. Make sure you get in a good cardiovascular workout at least three times a week for at least thirty minutes per session.

When I talk about *contracting your core,* I'm referring to the muscles from your upper chest to your thighs, primarily your abs. A strong core makes for better fitness, better posture, and more endurance. By contracting your core, I basically mean "pulling in your gut."

Stretch for a few minutes after each session—even if you say you don't have time. Stretching gives you more flexibility, improves circulation and posture, and helps with your balance and coordination. Stretching also increases your range of motion (ROM), the ability to, say, reach up to a high shelf in your kitchen or throw a ball or pick up a bag of groceries (without throwing out your back).

RECAP

Before we turn to the Power Moves workouts, let's just do a quick recap. Exercise is an essential component in your journey to transform your body and your life. The following Power Moves workouts are a great tool to get you started, and they include some of my very favorite exercises. These programs are intended to get you thinking about how and why certain movements will lead to certain results, and in particular how focusing on the basic motions of the four major joint groups—our shoulders, elbows, hips, and knees—will allow you to achieve a full-body workout.

In addition to these workouts, you will need to perform some form of cardio (walking is great) at least three times a week for at least half an hour. Cardio is an excellent (and essential) supplement to resistance training. There are three resistance-training workouts introduced in this section—the No-Excuses workout, the Maintain/Stay-in-the-Game workout, and the Warrior workout. Look at each one and decide which is best suited to you and your particular goals and needs. If in doubt, start with No-Excuses. If it seems too easy, you can always increase the intensity by adding more repetitions, or just going faster. And last but not least, don't forget to stretch!

A final note: Make sure you speak to your physician before starting this or any other exercise program.

The Workouts

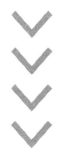

NO-EXCUSES WORKOUT

I created this workout for my clients who are always giving me excuses, the folks who:

- never have enough time to exercise.
- can't fit exercise into their hectic lives.
- travel on business and don't have room in their luggage for exercise equipment.
- don't know where to start.
- are afraid of injuring themselves.
- want to start out right—losing weight and getting toned the healthy way.

Do any of these sound like you?

Instructions: A complete No-Excuses workout should consist of one, two, or three sets of the selected routine. For example: Begin with the first exercise in your selected routine and continue through to the end, at which point you can begin again with the first exercise for your second set and repeat as above. If you choose to challenge yourself, you can continue on to a third set after the second round of exercises is complete. However, you should not feel confined to these routines. Once you get comfortable with the exercises you can think of different ways to mix them up and even create your own. These routines are just some good examples that I've come up with. But I encourage you to find what you enjoy best and continue to mix it up, by adding in other exercises you enjoy or by simply switching up the order and number of repetitions.

Repetitions: I always recommend beginning with a number that feels comfortable and working your way toward 12–15.

Time to complete: The No-Excuses workout should take less than 20 minutes *per set*.

Calories: The No-Excuses workout should burn approximately 175 calories per set. Keep in mind you will also benefit from EPOC (post-exercise calorie burn for up to fifteen hours).

Stretch time: You should do at least five minutes of stretching after the No-Excuses workout.

Joints engaged: The following icons will let you know which joints each exercise engages:

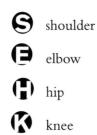 shoulder

elbow

hip

knee

SQUAT PRESS

Joints Engaged: Ⓢ Ⓗ Ⓔ Ⓚ

Muscles Worked: Primary–Quadriceps, Shoulders; Secondary–Hamstrings, Glutes, Core*

The squat press is an excellent exercise that can be done with body weight alone or with added weights.

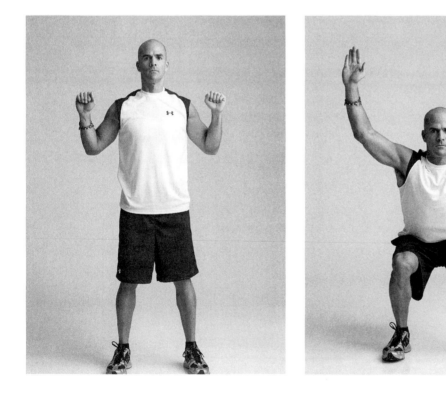

1. Stand with your feet shoulder width apart. Your arms should be bent with hands at shoulder height.

2. Squat down with your hips pushed back, as if you were about to sit in a chair.

3. Continue to squat until your thighs are parallel to the ground.

4. As you squat, simultaneously reach up with your arms toward the sky.

5. Slowly come back to starting position: standing with your hands at shoulder height.

6. Repeat. Begin with 5 and build up to 15 reps.

>>tips:

Keep your back straight and contract your core throughout the movement. Heels should *always* remain in contact with the ground.

*Core = the muscles of your abs and back, which support the spine.

REVERSE LUNGE PRESS

Joints Engaged: Ⓢ Ⓔ Ⓗ Ⓚ

Muscles Worked: Primary–Hamstrings, Quadriceps, Shoulders; Secondary–Glutes, Triceps, Core

The lunge is an excellent exercise to tone and shape your thighs, butt, and calves. Combining it with a press simultaneously tones and builds upper-body strength.

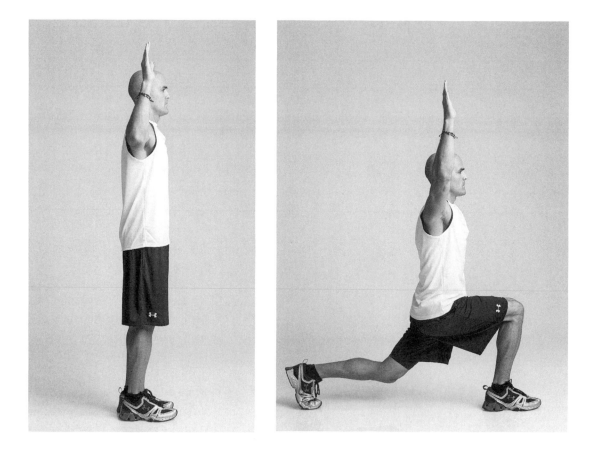

1. Stand with your feet shoulder width apart. Elbows are bent at shoulder height, palms facing front.

2. Step back with your left leg and reach your arms toward the sky.

3. At the same time, bend your right leg at the knee; your knee should be in line with your ankle–not your toes.

4. Return to starting position.

5. Repeat on right side.

6. Repeat both sides 5 times, building up to 15 reps.

>>**tips:**

Keep your back straight and core contracted throughout the movement. Hand weights can be added for increased resistance and greater results.

exercise 3

SINGLE-LEG AND PELVIC LIFT

Joints Engaged: (H) (K)

Muscles Worked: Primary–Hamstrings, Glutes; Secondary–Core

This is an excellent exercise for endurance and stability of the hamstrings and glutes.

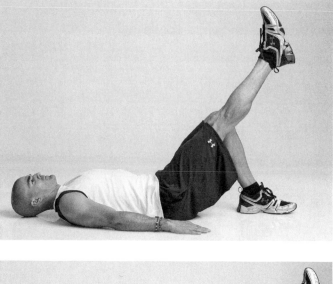

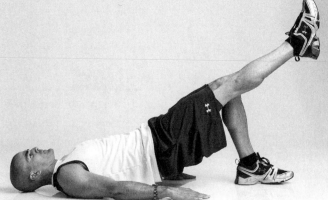

1. Lie down on your back.

2. Bend both knees and place the soles of your feet flat on the ground.

3. Extend and lift one leg while keeping it parallel to the other thigh.

4. Tighten your abdominal muscles by pulling in, as if a string in your back was pulling you.

5. Slowly lift your hips off the floor.

6. Repeat with other leg.

7. Repeat 5 times with both legs, building up to 15 reps.

>>tips:

Do not allow your glutes to touch the ground between repetitions.

PUSH-UP INTO SIDE PLANK

Joints Engaged: Ⓢ Ⓔ Ⓗ

Muscles Worked: Primary—Chest, Shoulders; Secondary—Triceps, Core, Oblique Abdominals

This is a new twist on a timeless classic: the push-up.

1. Begin in classic push-up position: feet together, hands placed firmly on the ground shoulder width apart, body slightly lifted in a straight line.

2. Lower your body, bending your elbows, until you are a few inches off the ground. Do not touch the ground.

3. Return to starting position and shift your body weight onto one arm.

4. Raise the other arm toward the sky and turn so you face forward in a plank position.

5. Bring the arm down. Slowly move back to starting position.

6. Repeat the push-up, and then switch arms for the plank.

7. Repeat 5 times on each side, building up to 15 reps.

>>tips:

Start off slowly until you develop the balance, coordination, and strength to go through the exercise without compromising your form. If you have difficulty performing a complete push-up, start by lowering yourself only halfway down to the floor, increasing the range as you get stronger.

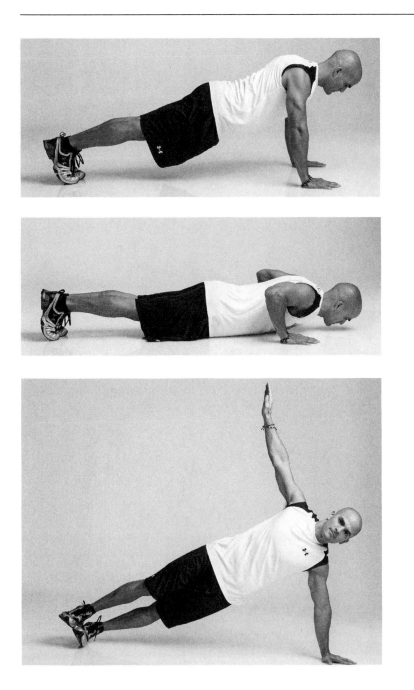

THE MODIFIED COBRA

Joints Engaged: Ⓢ Ⓔ Ⓗ Ⓚ

Muscles Worked: Primary–Lower Back; Secondary–Chest, Triceps, Shoulders, Core

A variation of the yoga posture used since ancient times.

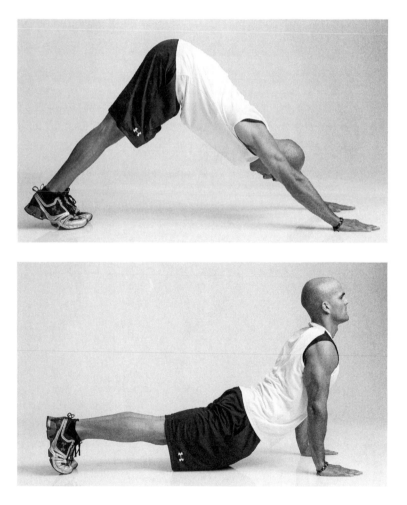

1. Start off in a push-up position: feet together, toes on the floor, hands placed firmly on the ground shoulder width apart, body slightly lifted in a straight line.

2. Stretch your shoulders out to the front, keeping your hands firmly on the ground.

3. Pull yourself up by the hips. Pretend there is a string pulling your hips up toward the sky. At the same time push your hips back without bending the knee. If you look in a mirror, your body would form a triangular shape.

4. Shift your body weight to the back as you slowly lower your body. Move your arms on either side of your shoulders, palms down, fingers facing front.

5. "Scoop" your upper body up as far as it will go **without any strain** as you return your bottom half to the start position. Make sure your arms are locked at the sides.

6. Gently bring your upper body to the floor, and then repeat.

7. Repeat 5 times, building up to 15 reps.

>>tips:

Keep your core contracted, your abdominal muscles tight, throughout this movement. Never pull yourself up to the point of straining.

exercise

6

REVERSE DIP

Joints Engaged: Ⓢ Ⓔ Ⓗ Ⓚ

Muscles Worked: Primary–Triceps; Secondary–Shoulders, Chest

If you are in a hotel room, an office, or at home, there's still no excuse: simply use a desk chair for this move. Make sure it is stabilized with its back to the wall or bed.

1. Place your hands on a bench (chair edge), hands facing front, elbows bent.

2. Lock your knees and lower your body toward the ground until your elbows are bent and your upper arms are parallel to the ground.

3. Slowly bring yourself back to starting position.

4. Repeat 5 times, building up to 15 reps.

>>tips:

For an extra power boost, keep one leg in the air throughout the exercise, changing legs with each rep.

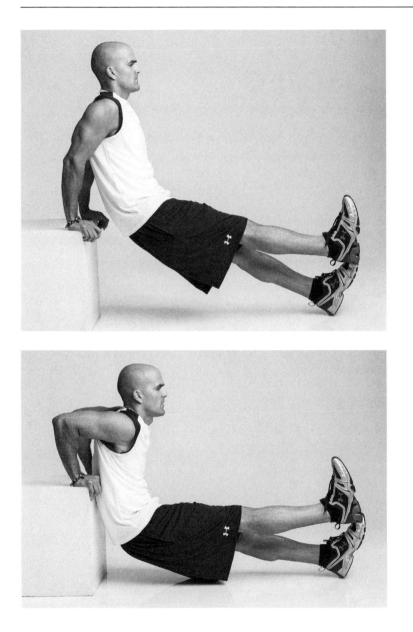

PIKE PUSH-UP

Joints Engaged: Ⓢ Ⓔ Ⓗ Ⓚ

Muscles Worked: Primary—Shoulders; Secondary—Triceps, Chest, Core

This is a classic push-up modified into a shoulder press. It is an incredible full-body exercise and yields amazing results!

1. Start in the classic push-up position (feet together, hands placed firmly on the ground shoulder width apart), but this time keep your feet on an elevated surface (a chair seat or piece of luggage).

2. Walk your hands back until your hips are higher than the rest of your body. Keep your back straight.

3. Bend the elbows and lower your body as if you were doing an inverted shoulder press. Your shoulders should bear the weight and your back should be straight.

4. Slowly return to starting position.

5. Repeat 5 times, building up to 15 reps.

>>tips:

Start with your upper and lower body forming a 45-degree angle. As you become stronger, you can work toward 90 degrees—the maximum stance.

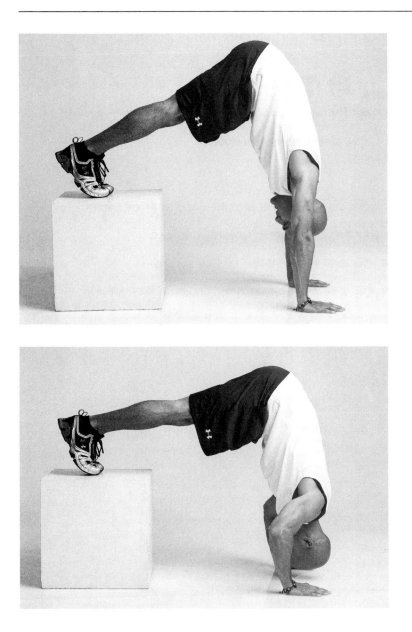

exercise

8

V-UPS

Joints Engaged: Ⓢ Ⓗ Ⓚ

Muscles Worked: Primary–Abdominals, Hip Flexors; Secondary–Lower Back

This is a great exercise for six-pack abs!

1. Lie down on your back, your feet together, and arms extended.

2. Pull up with your fingers reaching toward your toes.

3. At the same time, pull your feet up.

4. Try to touch your toes with your fingers, forming a V shape.

5. Slowly lower your legs and your arms to the starting position.

6. Repeat 10 times, building up to 25 reps.

>>tips:

Imagine you are balancing your body on your glutes as you touch toes and fingers.

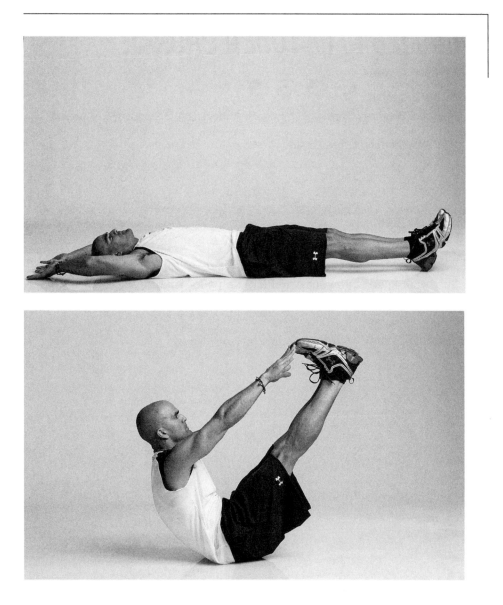

exercise
9

MODIFIED HEEL-TOUCH CRUNCH

Joints Engaged: Ⓢ Ⓔ Ⓗ Ⓚ

Muscles Worked: Primary–Hip Flexors, Abdominals; Secondary–Lower Back

Another great ab exercise!

1. Lie down on your back, your head and feet approximately six inches off the ground.

2. Sit up as high as possible.

3. Tuck your knees into your chest and reach for your heels.

4. Slowly unbend your knees and return to the starting position.

5. Repeat 10 times, building up to 25 reps.

>>tips:

Keep your feet together. Make sure your heels are in the same line with your hands: parallel to the ground.

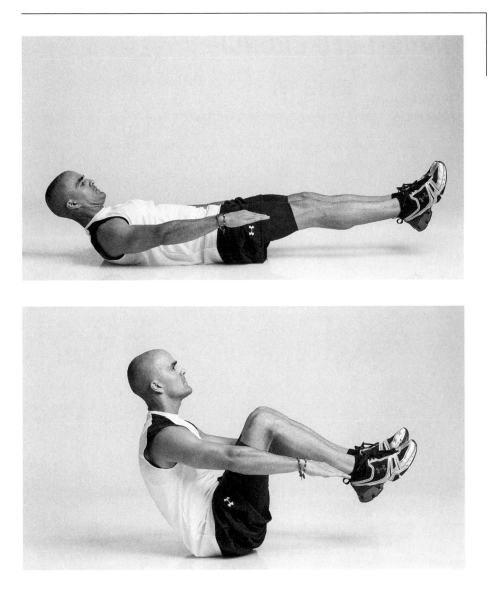

exercise

10

STRAIGHT-LEG CRUNCH

Joints Engaged: Ⓢ Ⓔ Ⓗ

Muscles Worked: Primary—Abdominals; Secondary—Hamstrings, Lower Back

Not only is this an excellent exercise for your abdominals, but it also gives your hamstrings a nice stretch.

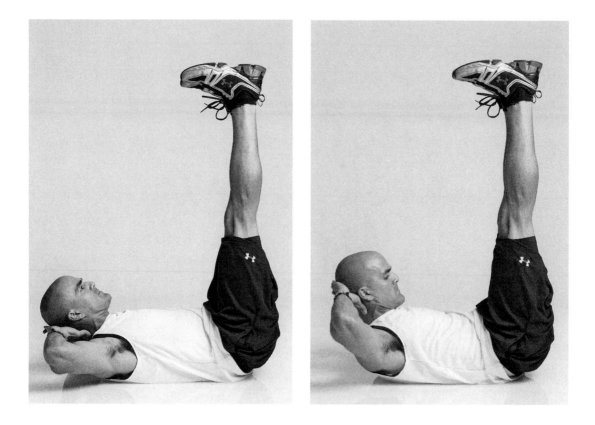

1. Lie down on your back with your legs locked and straight up in the air. (Imagine a hinge at your waist.) Hands should be firmly placed behind your head.

2. Slowly curl your back up toward your straight-up legs.

3. Slowly move back to the floor.

4. Repeat 10 times, building up to 25 reps, and return to starting position, controlling the movement throughout.

>>tips:

Use your hands to support your head only. Do not use your hands to pull your head up—it's bad for your neck (places too much pressure on the cervical spine)!

UPRIGHT BICYCLE CRUNCH

Joints Engaged: Ⓢ Ⓔ Ⓗ Ⓚ

Muscles Worked: Primary—Obliques; Secondary—Abdominals, Hip Flexors, Lower Back, Core

There's a reason the bicycle has been around for a long time—it's a great total core workout. I've added a twist to keep it new.

1. Sit on the floor, leaning back so that your body is balanced on your butt, knees are slightly bent, and feet are off the floor.

2. Place your hands beside your head with your elbows up and out.

3. Alternate touching each elbow to its opposite knee, keeping in a sitting position with your feet off the floor.

4. Repeat 10 times, building up to 25 reps (touching both sides equals one rep).

>>tips:

Keep one foot on the ground in the beginning until you develop the core strength to balance your body without touching the floor.

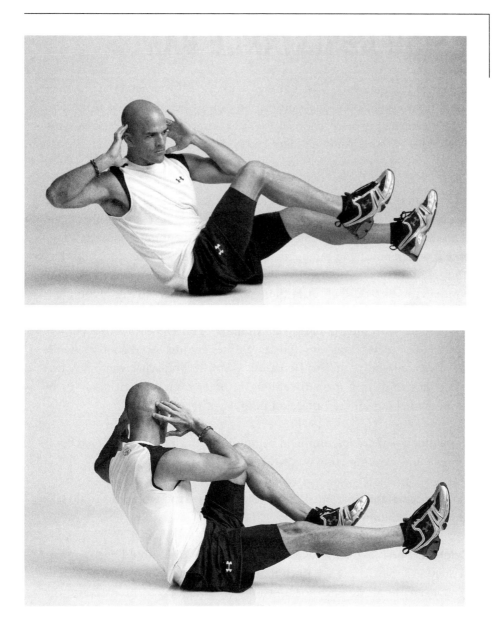

NO-EXCUSES WORKOUT USING RESISTANCE BANDS

This is a variation on my No-Excuses workout. All you need is a resistance band. If you don't own one, you can buy one, borrow one, or make one. It's a great thing to have. You can use it at home, at the gym, and you can even travel with it (it doesn't take up any room in a suitcase).

And remember, don't just resist—persist!

Instructions: A complete No-Excuses Resistance-Band workout should consist of one, two, or three sets of the selected routine. For example: Begin with the first exercise in your selected routine and continue through to the end, at which point you can begin again with the first exercise for your second set and repeat as above. If you choose to challenge yourself, you can continue on to a third set after the second round of exercises is complete. However, you should not feel confined to these routines. Once you get comfortable with the exercises you can think of different ways to mix them up and even create your own. These routines are just some good examples that I've come up with. But I encourage you to find what you enjoy best and continue to mix it up, by adding in other exercises you enjoy or by simply switching up the order and number of repetitions.

Repetitions: I always recommend beginning with a number that feels comfortable and working your way toward 12–15.

Time to complete: The No-Excuses Resistance-Band workout should take less than 20 minutes *per set*.

Calories: The No-Excuses Resistance-Band workout should burn approximately 175 calories per set. Keep in mind you will also benefit from EPOC (post-exercise calorie burn for up to fifteen hours).

Stretch time: You should do at least five minutes of stretching after the No-Excuses Resistance-Band workout.

Joints engaged: The following icons will let you know which joints each exercise engages:

S   shoulder

E   elbow

H   hip

K   knee

exercise

1

SHOULDER FLY LUNGE

Joints Engaged: Ⓢ Ⓔ Ⓗ Ⓚ

Muscles Worked: Primary–Quadriceps, Shoulders; Secondary–Hamstrings, Glutes, Core

Think of this as two for one: one exercise for both upper and lower body at the same time.

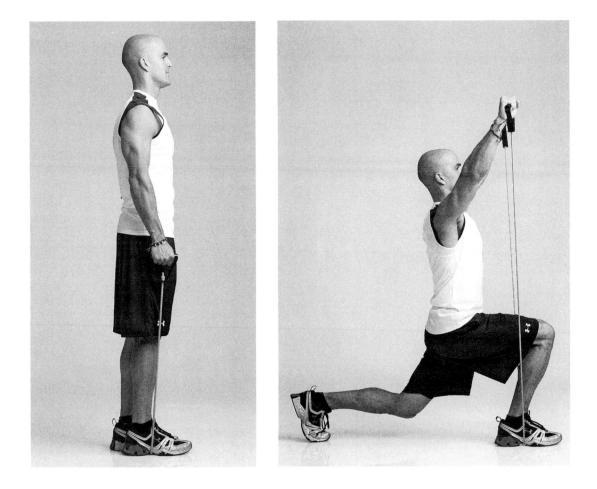

1. Begin with your feet shoulder width apart and resistance band securely under the foot that will be stationary. Hold band at your sides, palms facing in.

2. Step back (lunge) with the opposite foot (free foot without the band).

3. At the same time, quickly raise your arms using your shoulders.

4. Step forward. Lower arms.

5. Repeat with other foot.

6. Repeat 5 times with each foot, up to 15 reps.

>>tips:

Keep your moves fluid and continuous (one motion back, one motion up). It should feel like a simultaneous movement with both arms and legs.

exercise 2

REVERSE CHEST FLY

Joints Engaged: Ⓢ Ⓔ

Muscles Worked: Primary–Chest; Secondary–Shoulders, Core

This is one of the few great standing chest exercises.

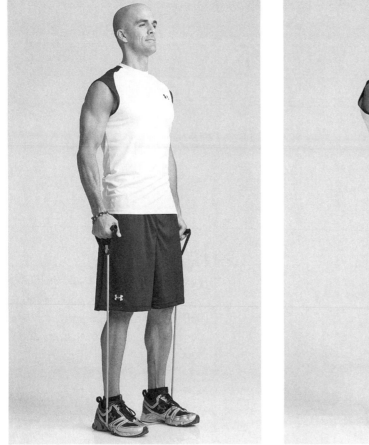

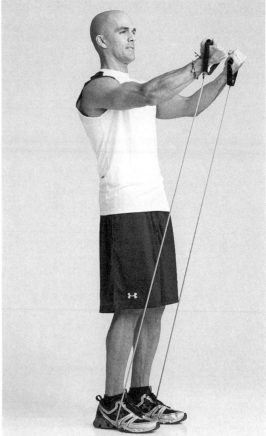

1. Stand with your feet shoulder width apart and with the band securely under the middle of both feet. Hold band at your sides, palms facing in.

2. Tighten your abs and, keeping a slight bend to your elbows, push the band (palms up) up to the height of your nose.

3. Lower your arms.

4. Repeat 5 times, building up to 15 reps.

>>tips:

Keep your back straight at all times.

exercise 3

ROWS

Joints Engaged: Ⓢ Ⓔ Ⓗ Ⓚ

Muscles Worked: Primary–Back; Secondary–Biceps, Rear Deltoids, Core

This is a great exercise to keep your back strong and to tone your arms.

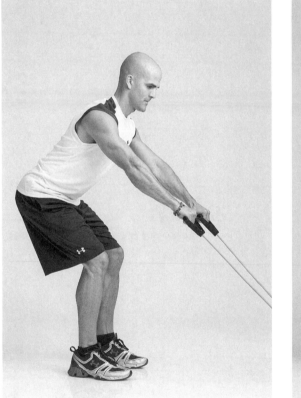
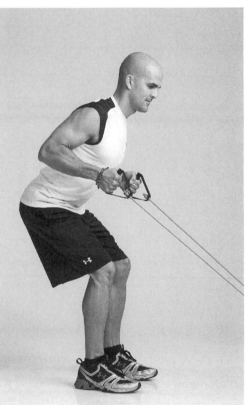

1. Begin with your feet shoulder width apart and the band securely fastened directly in front of you. (Use the knob of a closed door, a column, a gym pole, anything that's firmly in place.) Hold band with two hands.

2. Bend at the knees and lean forward slightly while keeping your back straight.

3. Pull the band toward the bottom of your chest.

4. Return to the starting position.

5. Repeat 5 times, building up to 15 reps.

>>tips:

Control the resistance throughout the entire motion; keep it steady.

exercise 4

BICEPS CURLS

Joints Engaged: E

Muscles Worked: Primary—Biceps; Secondary—Core

A simple way to tone and strengthen your biceps without expensive gym equipment.

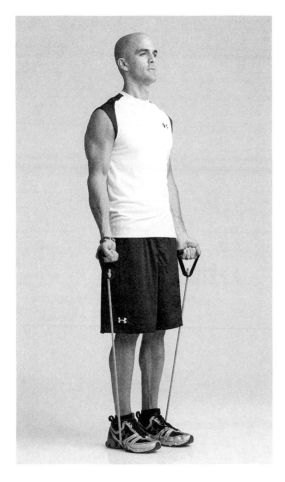

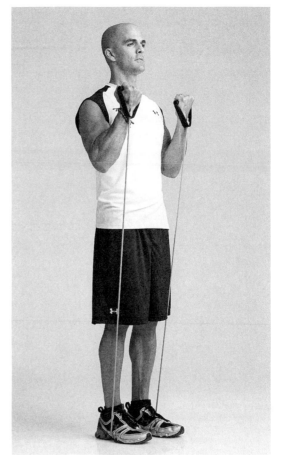

1. Begin with feet shoulder width apart and band securely fastened under the middle of both feet. Hold the band at your sides, palms facing forward.

2. Keeping your elbows at your sides, curl the band up to the tops of your shoulder.

3. Slowly lower the band to starting position.

4. Repeat 5 times, building up to 15 reps.

>>tips:

Keep your core contracted and back straight. Do not swing your body.

exercise 5

TRICEPS KICK

Joints Engaged: Ⓢ Ⓔ Ⓗ Ⓚ

Muscles Worked: Primary–Triceps; Secondary–Shoulders, Core

An old favorite kicks it up a notch.

1. Begin with one foot forward and one foot back. The band should be securely placed under the foot in the front. Hold the band with two hands.

2. Lean forward while keeping your back straight.

3. Move your elbows back slightly farther than your back. Your upper arms should be locked in place.

4. Using just your lower arms, push (kick) the band back until the elbow joint is almost at locked position. The upper arms do not move.

5. Return to starting position using only your triceps.

6. Repeat 5 times, building up to 15 reps.

>>tips:

Keep your movement controlled and smooth. Modify this move by fastening the band to a doorknob of a closed door or any other firmly planted object in front of you.

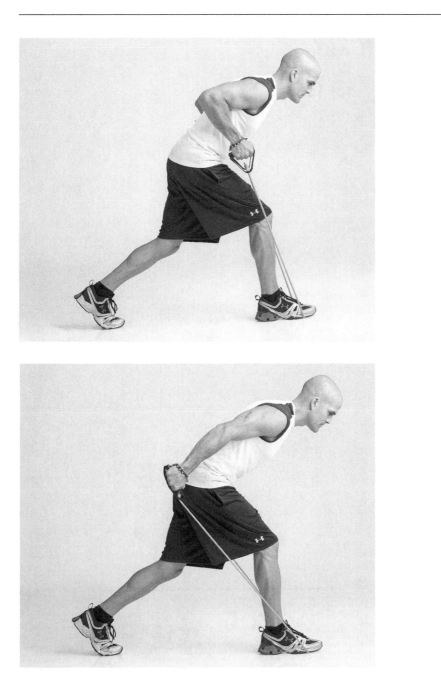

exercise 6

SHOULDER FLY

Joints Engaged: **S** **E**

Muscles Worked: Primary—Shoulders; Secondary—Core

This one is great for sculpting beautiful shoulders.

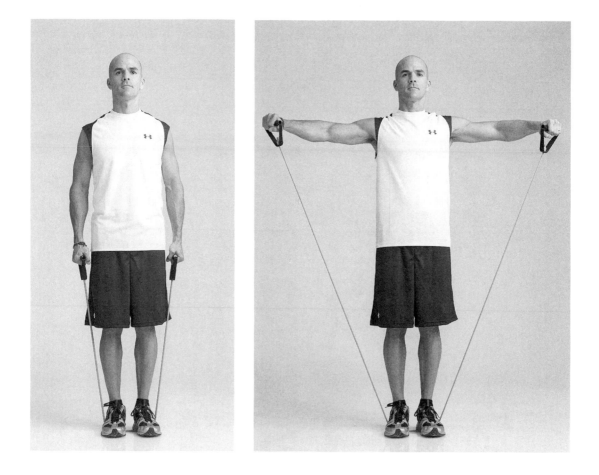

1. Begin with your feet slightly closer than shoulder width, the band under both feet. Hold the band at your sides with palms facing in.

2. With a slight bend in the elbow, lift your arms out to the side until they are parallel to the floor.

3. Bring your arms back to starting position.

4. Repeat 5 times, building up to 15 reps.

>>**tips:**

Keep your back straight and core contracted. Keep your movement controlled and smooth.

exercise 7

REVERSE CRUNCH

Joints Engaged: Ⓢ Ⓔ Ⓗ Ⓚ

Muscles Worked: Primary–Abdominals, Hip Flexors; Secondary–Lower Back, Obliques (the sides of your abdomen)

Double the work in half the time.

1. Sit on the floor with your feet together. Secure the resistance band to an object in front of you (a column, a gym pole, anything that is firm and stable). Put your feet in the band, stirrup style.

2. Lean back, keeping your heels off the floor.

3. Pull your knees to your chest. At the same time pull your feet toward your upper body.

4. Return to starting position.

5. Repeat 5 times, building up to 25 reps.

>>tips:

Start off with your heels resting on the ground until you develop the strength to keep them in the air.

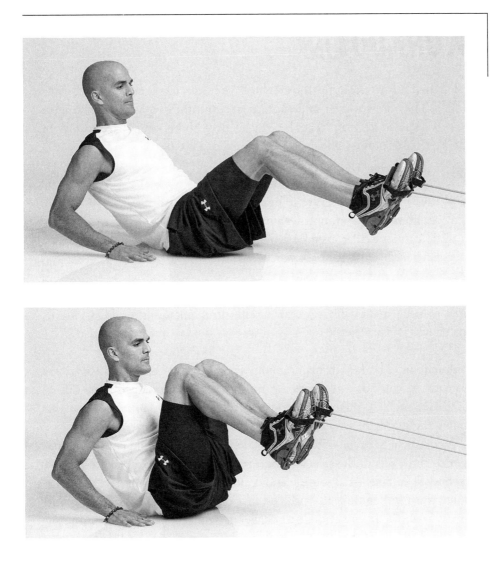

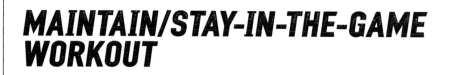

MAINTAIN/STAY-IN-THE-GAME WORKOUT

I designed this workout for those who have begun to see success with their bodies. They are stronger and more toned and they've lost some weight. But in order to keep up their healthy, fit new bodies, they have to rev up their exercise routine. This workout is for people who:

- have started or want to start losing weight.
- have incorporated exercise into their daily routine.
- are comfortable around weights and machines.
- do cardiovascular exercise at least three times a week.
- have more time to work out.

If you have set your short-term fitness and weight-loss goals, now it's time to keep it moving and concentrate on maintaining—and staying in the game.

Instructions: The key to maintaining/staying in the game is to vary your exercises so you don't get bored. In this spirit, I've introduced three different Maintain/Stay-in-the-Game workout options: #1, 2, and 3. You can follow them as they are presented, or you can mix and match.

A complete Maintain/Stay-in-the-Game workout should consist of one, two, or three sets of the selected routine. For example: Begin with the first exercise in your selected routine and continue through to the end, at which point you can begin again with the first exercise for your second set and repeat as above. If you choose to challenge yourself, you can continue on to a third set after the second round of exercises is complete. However, you should not feel confined to these routines. Once you get comfortable with the exercises you can think of different ways to mix them up and even create your own. These routines are just some good examples that I've come up with. But I encourage you to find what you enjoy best and continue to mix it up, by adding in other exercises you enjoy or by simply switching up the order and number of repetitions.

Repetitions: I always recommend beginning with a number that feels comfortable and working your way toward 12–15.

Time to complete: The Maintain/Stay-in-the-Game workout should take less than 30 minutes *per set*.

Calories: The Maintain/Stay-in-the-Game workout should burn approximately 250 calories per set. Keep in mind you will also benefit from EPOC (post-exercise calorie burn for up to fifteen hours).

Stretch time: You should do at least 10 minutes of stretching after the Maintain/Stay-in-the-Game workout.

Joints engaged: The following icons will let you know which joint each exercise engages:

S shoulder

E elbow

 H hip

 K knee

MAINTAIN/STAY-IN-THE-GAME WORKOUT Option #1

This plan uses a medicine ball, a bosu ball, a resistance ball and band, an incline bench, and dumbbells*—all standard equipment you can find in any gym. But if you're not near a gym, don't cop out. Try workout option #2 or 3, which use less equipment.

*Use weight that is easy enough for you to complete your set but challenging enough that you are not able to perform many more repetitions. For example, if you are doing sets of 10 reps, you want to be able to do all 10 reps but not 15 without it being a difficult challenge.

MAINTAIN/STAY-IN-THE-GAME WORKOUT Option #1

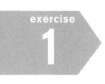

OVERHEAD MEDICINE BALL SQUAT

Joints Engaged: Ⓢ Ⓔ Ⓗ Ⓚ

Muscles Worked: Total Body

A fantastic exercise that works the whole body.

1. Begin with your feet shoulder width apart and the medicine ball between your palms overhead.

2. Drop down into a squat position while maintaining the medicine ball overhead. Your thighs should end up being parallel to the floor.

3. Contract your quads and bring yourself back to a standing position.

4. Repeat 10 times, building up to 15 reps.

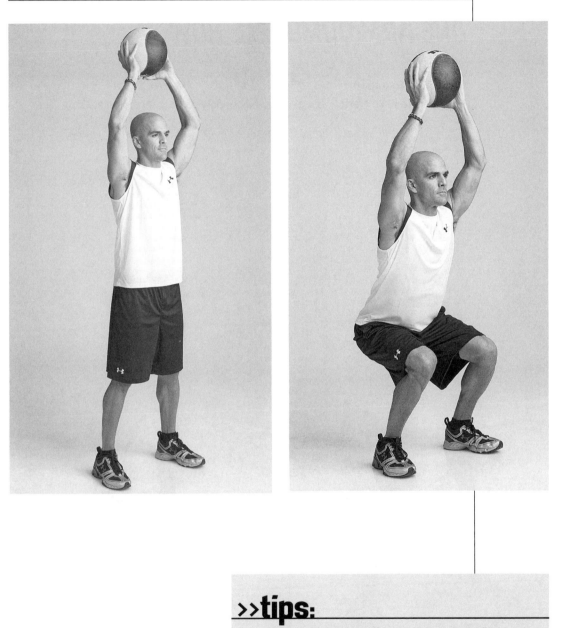

>>**tips:**

Keep your back straight and your abs pulled in.

exercise 2

ONE-ARM DUMBBELL ROW

Joints Engaged: Ⓢ Ⓔ Ⓗ Ⓚ

Muscles Worked: Primary–Back; Secondary–Biceps, Shoulders, Core

Great for back, arms, and core. Note to self: "Don't skip this one."

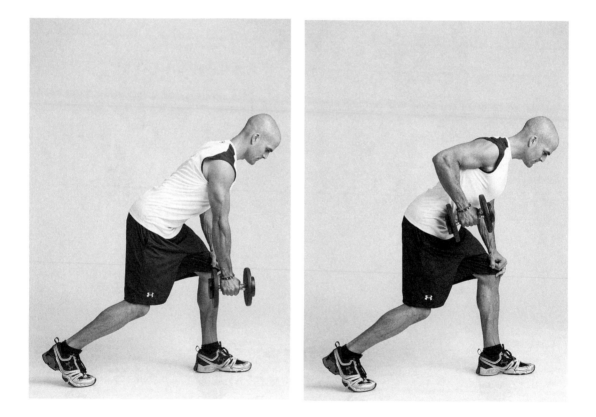

1. Begin with one foot forward and one foot back. Hold a dumbbell in the hand on the same side as the back foot; your arm should be perpendicular to the floor.

2. Pull the dumbbell up and slightly back until the weight reaches your lower chest.

3. Return to starting position.

4. Repeat 10 times, building up to 15 reps.

5. Repeat entire exercise with your other side.

6. Repeat 10 times, building up to 15 reps.

>>tips:

Keeping your abs tight helps keep your back straight. Start with a weight you can comfortably control until you've mastered the movement and it's no longer a challenge.

exercise 3

MEDICINE BALL LUNGE AND TWIST

Joints Engaged: **S** **E** **H** **K**

Muscles Worked: Primary—Quads, Obliques; Secondary—Hamstrings, Glutes, Shoulders, Core, Back, Biceps, and Triceps

This exercise is a favorite for many because of its ability to transform both glutes and gut.

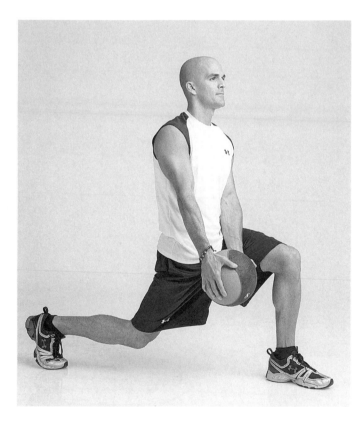

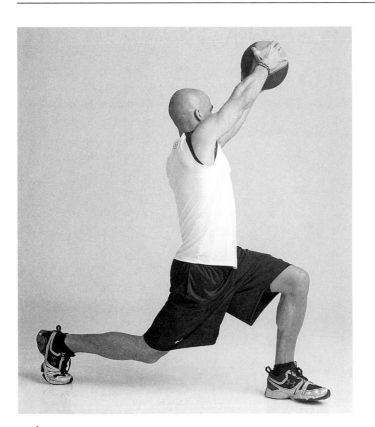

1. Begin with your feet shoulder width apart.

2. Lunge forward, holding the medicine ball in line with your body.

3. At the end of the lunge, reach up with the medicine ball and twist your trunk (core) across your forward leg.

4. Return, and repeat to the other side.

5. Repeat entire exercise 10 times, building up to 15 reps.

>>**tips:**

Keeping your ab muscles tight helps keep your back straight.

exercise 4

INCLINE CURL AND PRESS

Joints Engaged: Ⓢ Ⓔ Ⓗ Ⓚ

Muscles Worked: Primary—Chest, Biceps; Secondary—Shoulders, Triceps, Core

This exercise is a twofer—it targets biceps and chest.

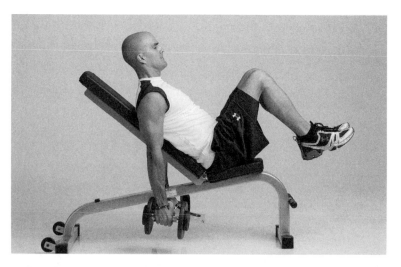

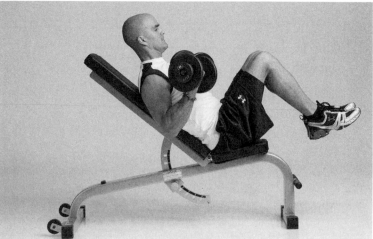

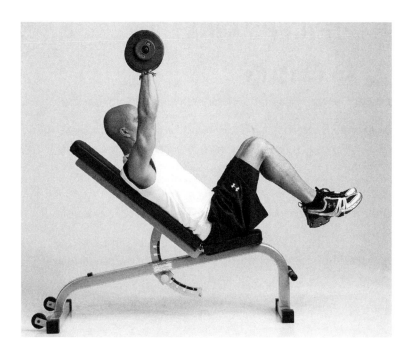

1. Lie flat on an incline bench with your knees up. Hold one dumbbell in each hand.

2. Curl the dumbbells up to the chest, then press up above your chest.

3. Bring the dumbbells back to your chest, then to the sides in the starting position.

4. Repeat 10 times, building up to 15 reps.

>>tips:

Keep your movement fluid and smooth from the first step through the last..

BOSU BALL TRICEPS KICK

Joints Engaged: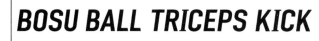

Muscles Worked: Primary—Triceps; Secondary—Shoulders, Core, Back

A great upper-body workout, especially good for core strength and stability. (A bosu ball provides an unstable surface for increased core stability.)

1. Sit up straight on a bosu ball (if you don't have one, sit on a couple of folded towels).

2. Bend your arms at the elbows and grip the cable pulley, stabilized resistance band, or rope behind your head.

3. Push your arms up straight toward the sky, keeping your elbows close to your head.

4. Bend back to starting position.

5. Repeat 10 times, building up to 15 reps.

>>tips:

Keeping your ab muscles tight helps keep your back straight. Keep your elbows in, close to the body.

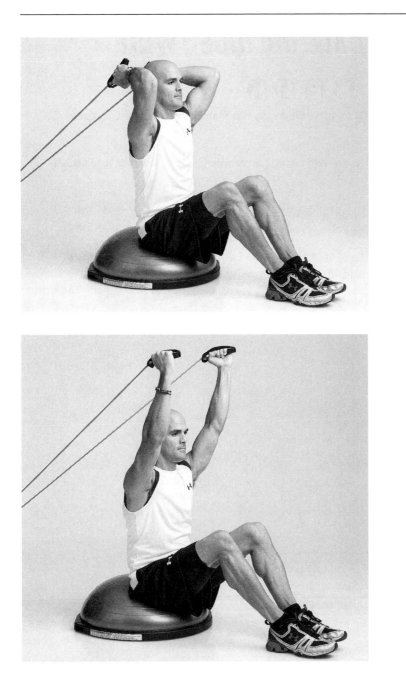

exercise 6

MEDICINE BALL OBLIQUE TWIST

Joints Engaged: Ⓢ Ⓔ Ⓗ Ⓚ

Muscles Worked: Primary–Obliques, Hip Flexors; Secondary–Shoulders, Core, Back, Biceps

The medicine ball adds extra resistance. Great for balance and stability.

1. Sit on the ground with your heels up and the medicine ball in both hands.

2. Turn your torso and touch the opposite knee with your elbow.

3. Repeat on the other side.

4. Alternate movement 10 times on each side, building up to 20 reps.

>>tips:

If you have trouble balancing with your heels in the air, keep them on the ground until you are stronger. A good way to ensure your heels stay up is to find a rhythm that works for you and stick to it as you move from side to side.

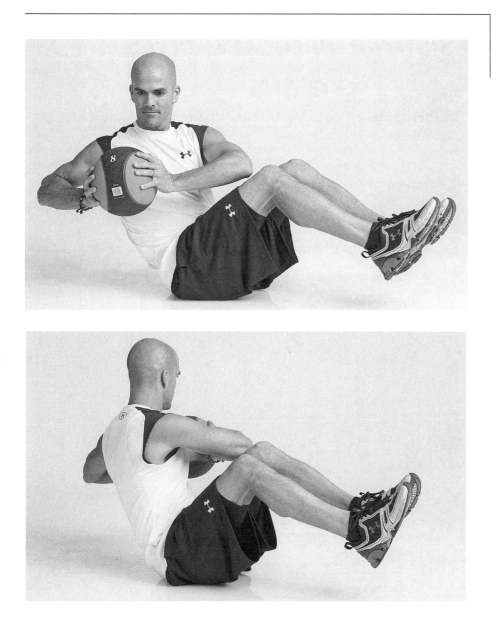

RESISTANCE-BALL JACKKNIVES

Joints Engaged: Ⓢ Ⓔ Ⓗ Ⓚ

Muscles Worked: Primary–Abs, Hip Flexors; Secondary–Obliques, Back, Shoulders, Biceps, Chest, Triceps

A challenging take on the classic push-up that gives the muscles of your upper body a great workout.

1. Begin in a classic push-up position with your feet on the resistance ball.

2. Quickly tuck your knees into your chest as you roll the ball in toward you.

3. Return to starting position.

4. Repeat 10 times, building up to 20 reps.

>>tips:

The trick to balancing your legs on the ball is keeping your core engaged throughout the movement.

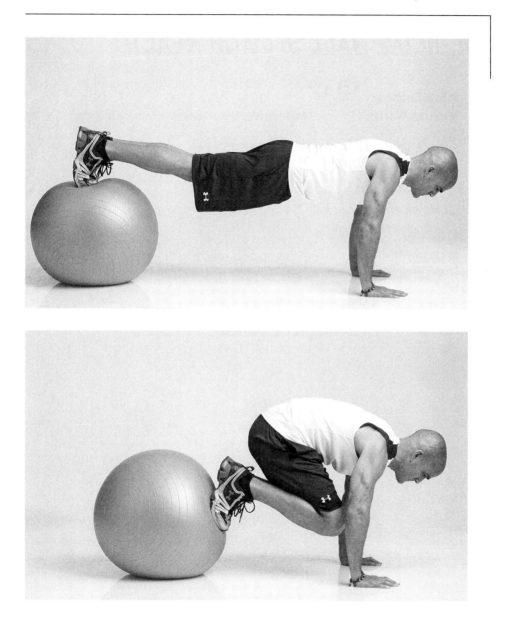

MEDICINE BALL SIT AND REACH

Joints Engaged: Ⓢ Ⓗ

Muscles Worked: Primary–Abdominals; Secondary–Shoulders, Triceps

An interesting twist on the standard sit-up.

1. Lie down on the floor with the medicine ball over your shoulders and your knees slightly bent.

2. In one explosive movement, sit up and reach to the sky with the medicine ball . . .

3. . . . and immediately return to the start position.

4. Repeat 10 times, building up to 20 reps.

>>tips:

Keep your arms perpendicular to the floor at all times.

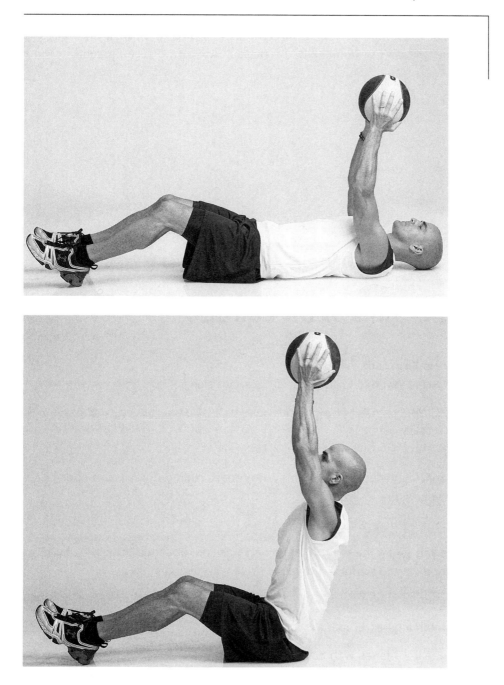

MAINTAIN/STAY-IN-THE-GAME WORKOUT Option #2

This plan uses a minimum of gym equipment: a medicine ball, a resistance ball and band, and a set of dumbbells. You may already own this equipment.

exercise 1

FRONT AND BACK LUNGE

Joints Engaged: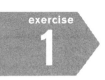

Muscles Worked: Primary–Quadriceps, Hamstrings, Glutes; Secondary–Core

With or without weights, this movement will keep your legs and glutes looking great!

1. Begin with your feet shoulder width apart. Hold a dumbbell in each hand at your sides, palms in.

2. Lunge forward with one leg.

3. As you return the leg to the starting position, continue through without stopping and perform a reverse lunge with the same leg.

4. Return to starting position.

5. Switch legs and repeat.

6. Repeat 10 times with each leg, going up to 15 reps.

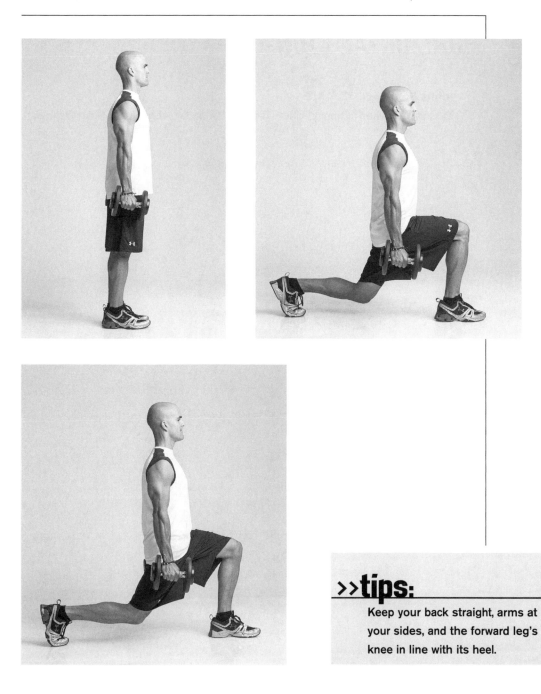

>>tips:

Keep your back straight, arms at your sides, and the forward leg's knee in line with its heel.

exercise 2

HORIZONTAL CHIN-UP

Joints Engaged: 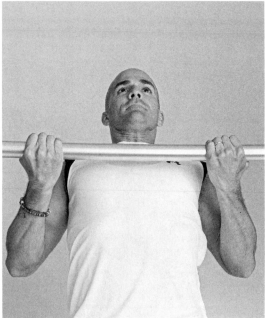 **S** **E**

Muscles Worked: Primary–Back, Biceps; Secondary–Shoulders (Rear Deltoids), Core

This is an alternative to the classic chin-up.

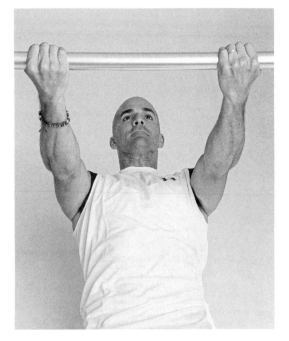

1. Lie on your back. Hold a bar with your palms facing your body and your hands slightly wider than shoulder width apart. Your feet should be together with heels resting on the floor.

2. Pull yourself toward the bar until it touches the top of your chest.

3. Slowly return to starting position.

4. Repeat 10 times, going up to 15 reps.

>>tips:

Keep your back straight by pulling in your abdominals. The more horizontal you get, the greater the resistance.

SPIDER MAN PUSH-UP

Joints Engaged: **S** **E** **H** **K**

Muscles Worked: Primary–Chest, Triceps; Secondary–Shoulders, Obliques, Hip Flexors

Classic push-up times ten!

1. Begin in classic push-up position: feet together, hands placed firmly on the ground shoulder width apart, body slightly lifted in a straight line.

2. Move one knee outside to the same line as your elbow.

3. Press down, keeping the knee in the "elbow position."

4. Come back up to start position and switch sides.

5. Repeat 10 times with each leg, up to 15 reps.

>>tips:

For more intensity, try doing all the repetitions to one side before switching to the other.

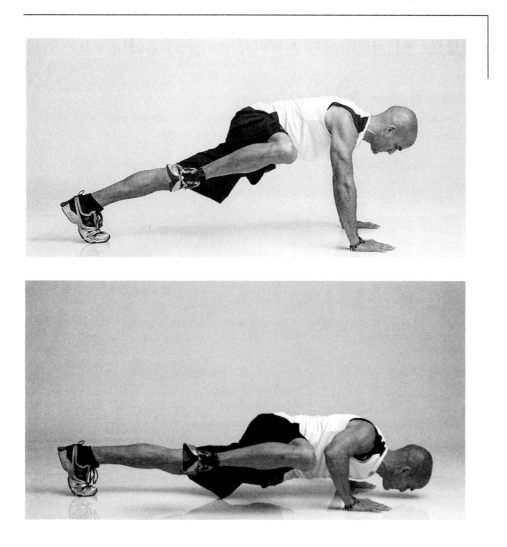

GOOD MORNING SINGLE-LEG LIFT

Joints Engaged: Ⓢ Ⓗ Ⓚ

Muscles Worked: Primary–Hamstrings, Lower Back; Secondary–Core, Shoulders

Stability, balance, and core strength all in one easy (looking) move.

1. Stand tall, your feet shoulder width apart, and your arms reaching up to the sky, close to your body.

2. Reach forward with your arms and body as one, as if there were a hinge at your waist.

3. Lift one leg off the ground while balancing on the other until your body is parallel to the floor.

4. Hold for a second, then come back to starting position.

5. Switch legs.

6. Repeat exercise with both legs 10–15 times.

>>tips:

Perform this movement slowly and with control. Keep your core stable and steady.

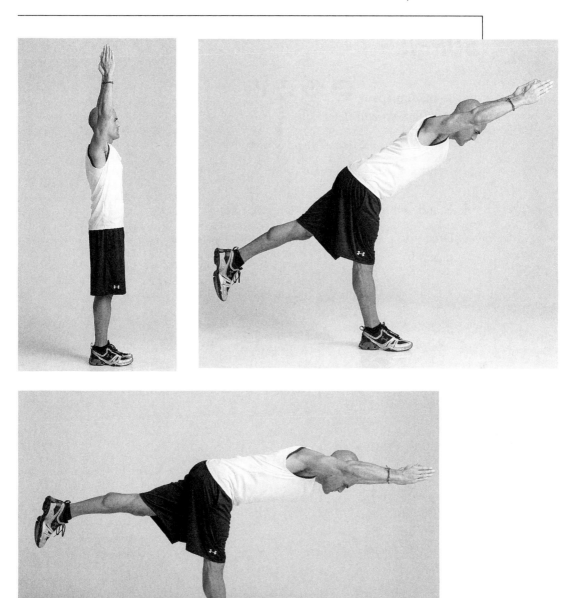

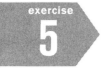

exercise

5

BURPIES

Joints Engaged: Ⓢ Ⓔ Ⓗ Ⓚ

Muscles Worked: Total Body

WOW, anyplace, anytime. Just try it.

1. Stand with your feet shoulder width apart.

2. Drop into a squat, your arms in front of you, your palms flat on the ground.

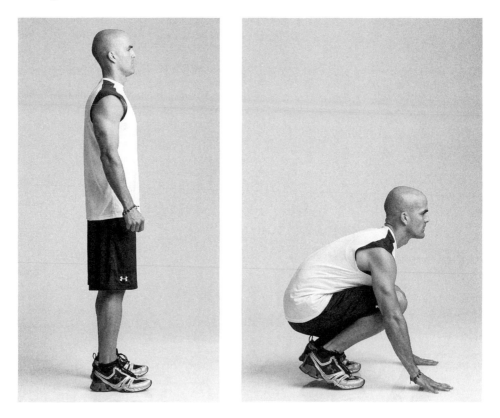

3. Thrust your feet back into a push-up position and complete one.

4. Thrust your feet back to the squat position.

5. Stand.

6. Repeat 10 times, going up to 20 reps.

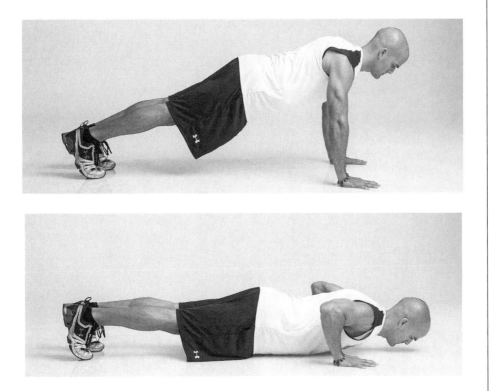

>>**tips:**

For a greater challenge, finish the
move with an explosive jump as
you get up from the squat to stand.

PLANK

Joints Engaged: Ⓢ Ⓔ Ⓗ Ⓚ

Muscles Worked: Primary–Core; Secondary–Shoulders, Triceps

How long can you hold this move? Ten seconds, thirty, a minute? Try it, record your results, and try it again in a month.

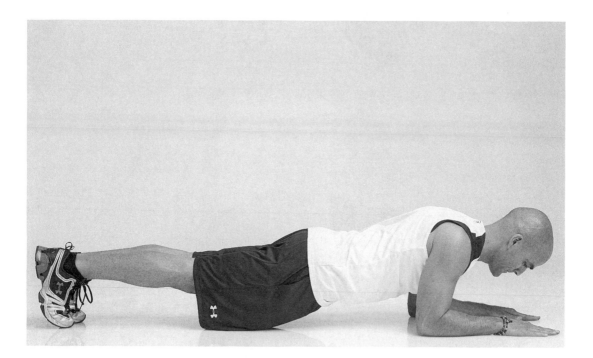

1. Begin in a classic push-up position (feet together, hands placed firmly on the ground shoulder width apart, body slightly lifted in a straight line).

2. Drop down to your elbows; your lower arms should be flat on the floor, hands facing out. Your hips should be in line with your body.

3. Hold this pose for a count of 10. Then relax.

4. Repeat 3 times.

>>tips:

For a greater challenge, try lifting one leg then switch to the other, as you hold the pose.

MEDICINE BALL SIT-UP TOUCH

Joints Engaged: Ⓢ Ⓔ Ⓗ Ⓚ

Muscles Worked: Primary–Abdominals; Secondary–Shoulders, Lower Back, Biceps

Builds explosiveness in the core, which is increasingly important as we get older.

1. Lie on your back on the floor with your knees bent and your arms extended. Grasp a medicine ball with your hands.

2. Quickly sit up, keeping your hands on the ball.

3. Keep moving forward until the medicine ball touches the floor between your feet.

4. Move back to starting position.

5. Repeat 10 times, building up to 20 reps.

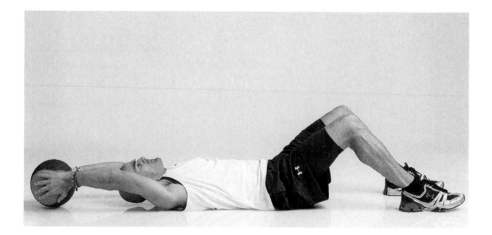

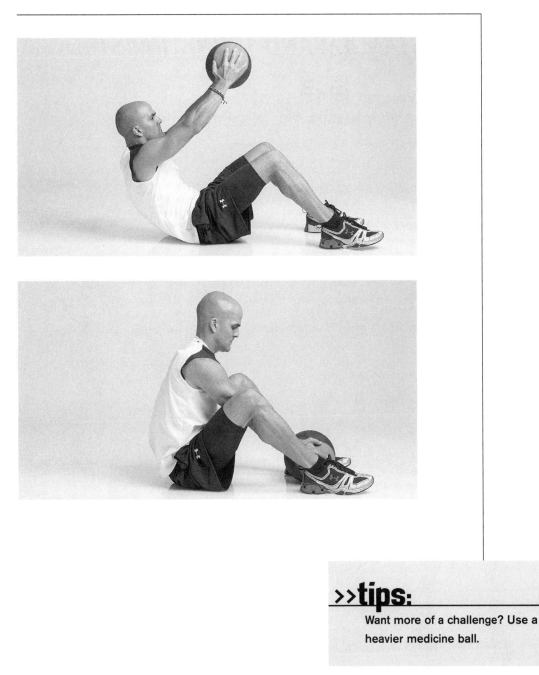

>>tips:

Want more of a challenge? Use a heavier medicine ball.

exercise

8

RESISTANCE-BAND TRUNK TWIST

Joints Engaged: Ⓢ Ⓔ

Muscles Worked: Primary–Core; Secondary–Shoulders, Triceps

Great move for core strength and stability.

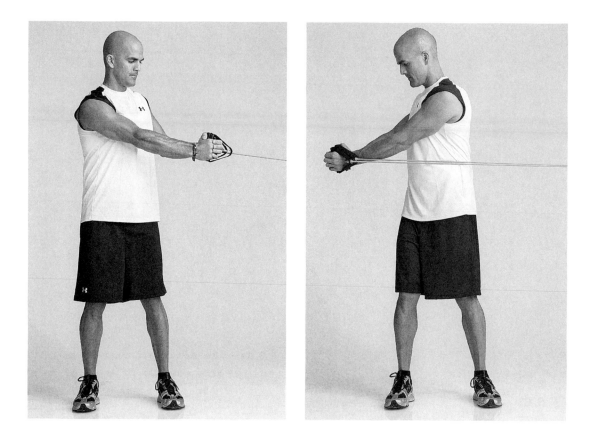

1. Stand with your feet shoulder width apart. Secure a resistance band around a fixed object or use a cable pulley. Hold handles with both hands in front of your body.

2. Without moving your lower body, twist your upper body away from the band—which remains solidly in front of you.

3. Twist to one side for all repetitions and then switch to the other side.

4. Repeat 10 times on each side, building up to 25 reps.

>>tips:

Keep your back straight and your abs tight for maximum results.

MAINTAIN/STAY-IN-THE-GAME WORKOUT Option #3

This variation uses barbells, dumbbells, and medicine balls. It's a way to Maintain/Stay in the Game—and enjoy it, too. Congratulations. You can work the gym with the best of them!

MAINTAIN/STAY-IN-THE-GAME WORKOUT Option #3

JUMPING LUNGE

Joints Engaged: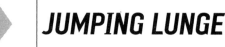

Muscles Worked: Primary–Quadriceps, Hamstrings; Secondary–Core

All the benefits of the classic lunge with added explosiveness (improves reaction time).

1. Begin in a lunge position, using either side. (One leg forward, knee bent and in line above foot; the other leg back, foot facing forward, knee almost touching the ground.)

2. Explosively jump to the opposite-side lunge.

3. Jump back. Repeat.

4. Do 10 times on each side, building up to 20 reps.

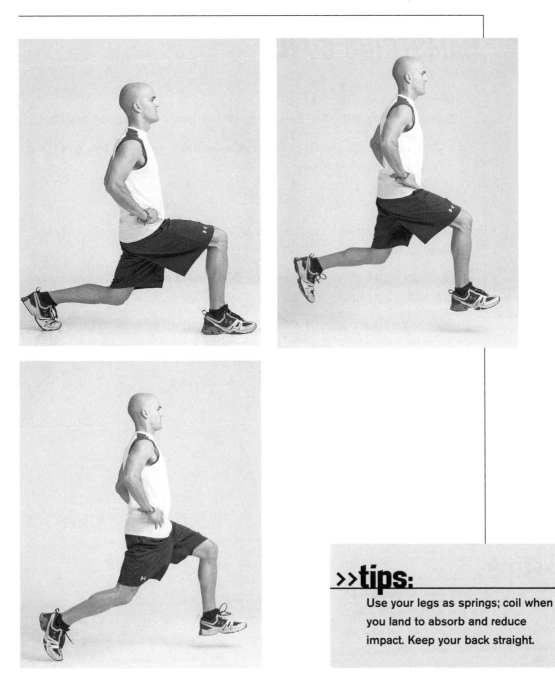

>>tips:

Use your legs as springs; coil when
you land to absorb and reduce
impact. Keep your back straight.

exercise 2

HAMSTRING CURL

Joints Engaged: **H** **K**

Muscles Worked: Primary—Hamstrings, Glutes; Secondary—Quadriceps, Core

Most people neglect their hamstrings. Here is a way to not only give them but get them the attention they deserve.

1. Lie on your back with one foot up on a resistance ball, the other slightly elevated above.

2. Contract your hamstrings (the back thighs) and roll the ball toward your butt with your foot.

3. Roll the ball back out until both legs are straight again.

4. Switch sides and repeat.

5. Do 8 times on each side, building up to 20 reps.

>>tips:

Beginners can start with both feet on the ball and work toward doing single-leg sets as they get stronger.

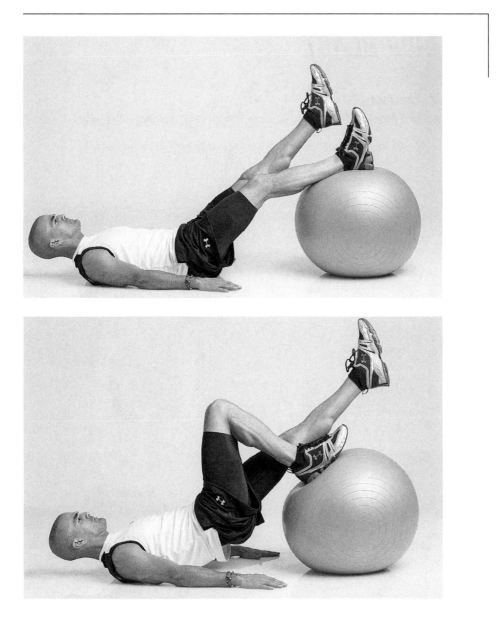

PULL-UP BLAST

Joints Engaged: Ⓢ Ⓔ Ⓗ Ⓚ

Muscles Worked: Primary—Back, Core; Secondary—Biceps, Hip Flexors

The extra move on this ordinary pull-up makes it extraordinary.

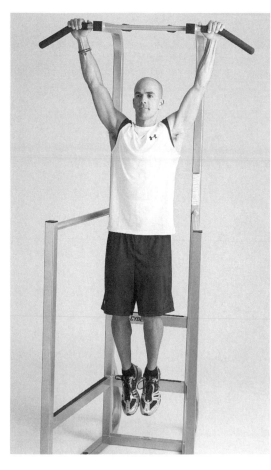

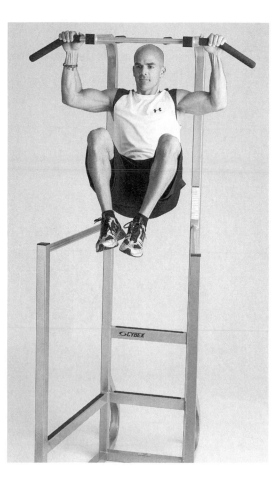

1. Begin in classic pull-up position (hands a bit wider than shoulder width).

2. In one explosive movement, pull yourself up and tuck your knees into your chest at the same time.

3. Control the movement as you return to start position and repeat.

4. Repeat 10 times, building up to 20 reps.

>>tips:

Keep your body stable; don't swing.

exercise 4

RESISTANCE-BALL CHEST PRESS

Joints Engaged: Ⓢ Ⓔ Ⓗ Ⓚ

Muscles Worked: Primary–Chest; Secondary–Triceps, Core

The resistance ball provides an unstable surface for greater core stability.

1. Place your back on the resistance ball, your legs bent, feet on the ground. Position yourself so that only your upper body is supported by the ball.

2. Slowly press the dumbbells over your chest until your elbows are almost locked.

3. Return to starting position.

4. Repeat 10 times, building up to 15.

>>tips:

For better balance, keep your back straight and pull in your abs.

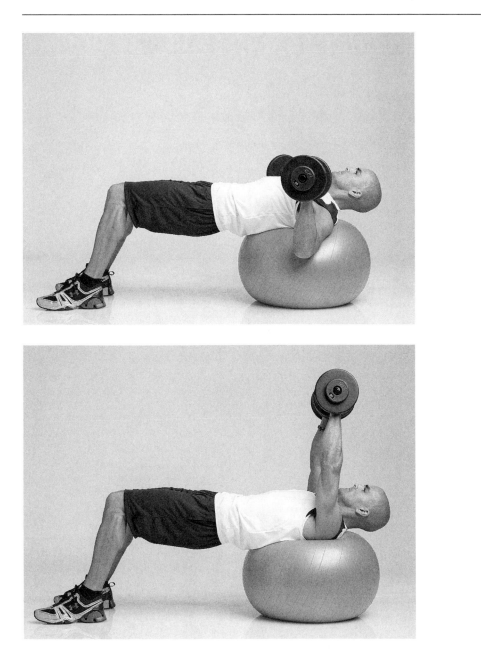

exercise 5

REVERSE-GRIP BARBELL CURL

Joints Engaged: E

Muscles Worked: Primary–Biceps; Secondary–Forearms, Shoulders

Great for toning not just biceps but also forearms.

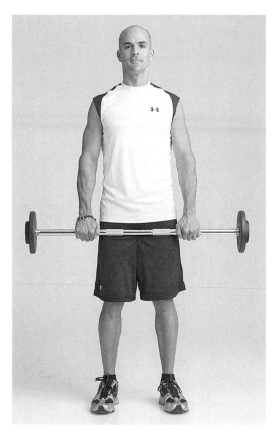

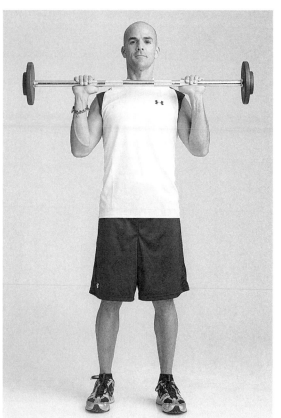

1. Stand tall, your feet shoulder width apart. Grasp a barbell, palms facing down, slightly wider than shoulder width. Your arms should be close to the sides of your body.

2. Curl the barbell up to the top of your chest, just under your neck.

3. Return to starting position.

4. Repeat 10 times, building up to 15 reps.

>>tips:

Keep your back straight, abdominals pulled in. Keep your body stable; don't swing.

exercise

6

OVERHEAD DUMBBELL EXTENSION

Joints Engaged: **S** **E**

Muscles Worked: Primary–Triceps; Secondary–Shoulders, Core

This exercise tones and defines the triceps.

1. Begin with your feet shoulder width apart. Grasp a dumbbell with your right hand; your free arm should be at your side.

2. Lift the dumbbell until your arm is fully extended over you.

3. Bend your elbow and lower the dumbbell behind your head.

4. In an arclike movement, raise the dumbbell back until your arm is fully extended and repeat.

5. Repeat 10 times, building up to 15 reps.

6. Switch sides.

>>tips:

Keep your back straight and
abdominals pulled in.

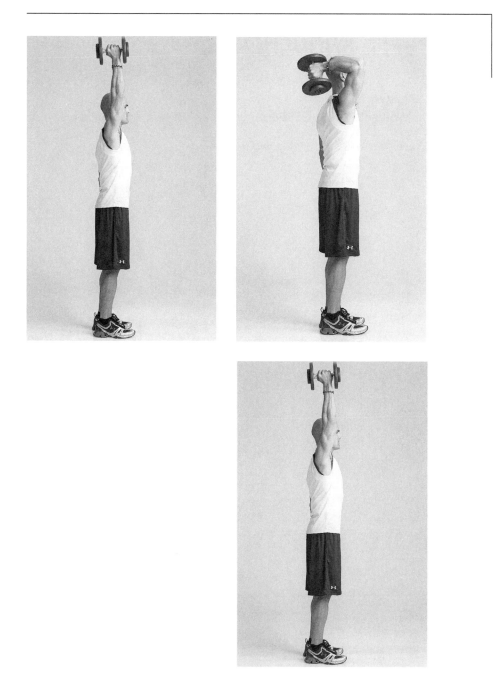

exercise
7

DUMBBELL SHOULDER FLY

Joints Engaged: Ⓢ Ⓔ

Muscles Worked: Primary–Shoulders; Secondary–Biceps, Trapezius, Core

Keeps your shoulders strong and pain-free.

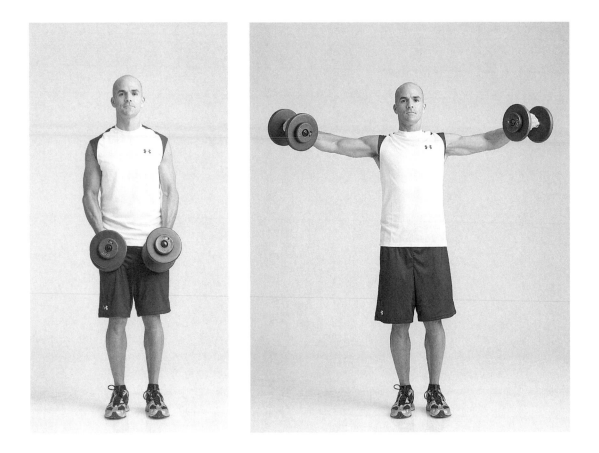

1. Stand tall, stomach in, and buttocks pulled in. Grasp a dumbbell in each hand, close to your sides, palms facing in.

2. Slowly raise the dumbbells outward until they are in line with the top of your shoulders.

3. Pause for a second, then slowly lower your arms to the starting position.

4. Repeat 10 times, building up to 15 reps.

>>**tips:**

Keep your back straight and your abdominals contracted. Your fists, grasping the dumbbells, should be parallel to the floor when you reach your shoulder line.

exercise

8

OBLIQUE SIDE PLANK

Joints Engaged: Ⓢ Ⓔ

Muscles Worked: Primary–Obliques; Secondary–Lower Back, Shoulders, Triceps

Builds incredible core strength.

1. Begin on your side in a plank position (one hand flat on the ground, holding your upper body up; feet one on top of the other, straight-legged; head in line with your body).

2. Raise the free arm up to the sky.

3. Using your obliques (on the sides of your abdomen), drop your hip to the floor, as close to the ground as possible without straining.

4. Contract your obliques and return to starting plank position.

5. Repeat 10 times, then switch to the other side.

6. Build up to 20 reps on each side.

>>tips:

Beginners may want to start by resting their elbow on the ground and work their way up to a fully extended arm.

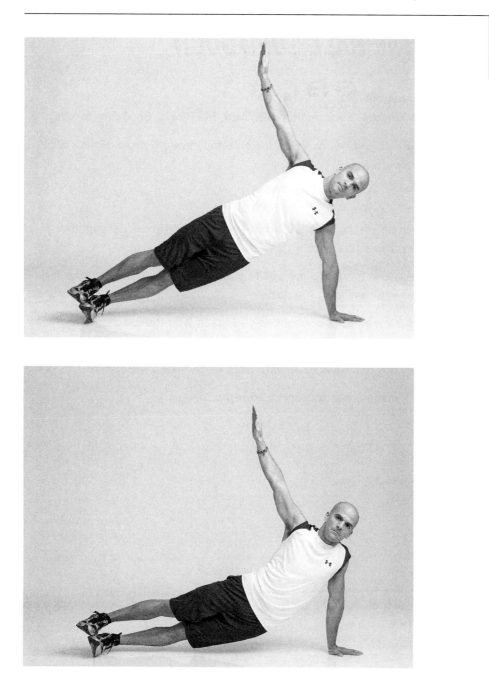

MEDICINE BALL TOE TOUCH

Joints Engaged: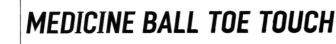

Muscles Worked: Abdominals, Lower Back, Hip Flexors, Shoulders, Biceps

This modified crunch works the core and develops balance and stability as well.

1. Begin seated on the floor with your knees up and your feet together. Grip a medicine ball in your hands.

2. Lean back with the medicine ball to your chest and straighten your legs as you lift your heels off the floor.

3. Bring your knees to your chest as you reach with the medicine ball toward your toes.

4. Return to position number 2 with heels off the floor and repeat.

5. Repeat 10 times, building up to 20 reps.

>>tips:

Your knees and upper body move toward each other simultaneously in a fluid, smooth motion.

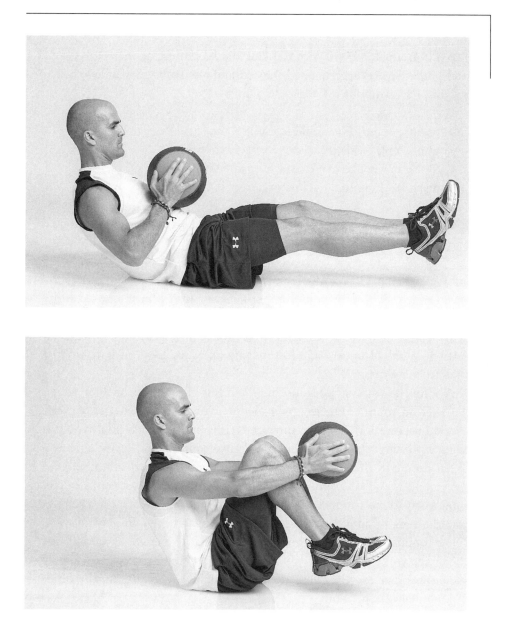

WARRIOR WORKOUT

This is for athletes, the top of the line, the workouts for those folks who have pushed up, sat up, crunched, pressed, and lifted with increasingly heavy weights. This workout is for people who:

- want to train for an athletic event.
- want to play a better game, whatever the sport.
- do cardiovascular exercise at least three times a week.
- make working out a priority.

If this sounds like you, go for it! You too can be a warrior, ready to take on the world.

Instructions: These two Warrior workout options are designed for experienced athletes who want to push their personal best, who want to beat the competition, who want to be strong, stay strong, and feel strong regardless of their age. Feel free to mix these workouts; just make sure you get in equal amounts of upper- and lower-body exercises. Do you have what it takes to be a warrior?

A complete Warrior workout should consist of one, two, or three sets of the selected routine. For example: Begin with the first exercise in your selected routine and continue through to the end, at which point you can begin again with the first exercise for your second set and repeat as above. If you choose to challenge yourself, you can continue on to a third set after the second round of exercises is complete. However, you should not feel confined to these routines. Once you get comfortable with the exercises you can think of different ways to mix them up and even create your own. These routines are just some good examples that I've come up with. But I encourage you to find what you enjoy best and continue to mix it up, by adding in other exercises you enjoy or by simply switching up the order and number of repetitions.

Repetitions: I always recommend beginning with a number that feels comfortable and working your way toward 12–15.

Time to complete: The Warrior workout should take less than 45 minutes *per set*.

Calories: The Warrior workout should burn approximately 450 calories per set. Keep in mind you will also benefit from EPOC (post-exercise calorie burn for up to fifteen hours).

Stretch time: You should do at least 10 minutes of stretching after the Warrior workout.

Joints engaged: The following icons will let you know which joint each exercise engages:

S shoulder

E elbow

H hip

K knee

WARRIOR WORKOUT Option #1

The gym is your element in this Warrior workout. Keep dumbbells, a barbell, a bosu ball, a medicine ball, a resistance ball, and even a towel nearby (if you sweat a lot, grab two towels).

WARRIOR WORKOUT Option #1

exercise 1

DEAD LIFT HIGH PULL

Joints Engaged: Ⓢ Ⓔ Ⓗ Ⓚ
Muscles Worked: Total Body

Builds explosiveness and total-body strength.

1. Begin with your feet shoulder width apart and your grip on the barbell slightly wider.

2. Drop your hips back as you would in a squat. The movement begins at the bottom position.

3. Drive your hips and the bar up at the same time. As you lift the bar into the movement keep your elbows higher than your hands and finish the motion at the top of the chest.

4. Control the weight as you return to the start position.

5. Repeat 10 times, building up to 15 reps.

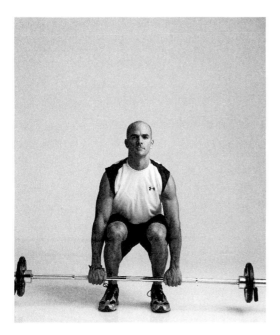
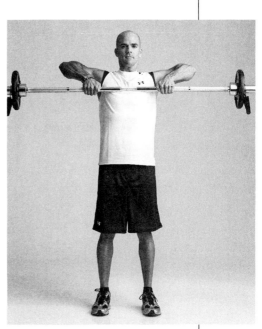

>>tips:

This move should be one fluid motion from start to finish. Keep your back straight and your core engaged throughout.

exercise

2

SINGLE-LEG DEAD LIFT

Joints Engaged: Ⓢ Ⓗ Ⓚ

Muscles Worked: Primary–Hamstring, Glutes; Secondary–Core

Targets the hamstrings and glutes but also develops balance and coordination.

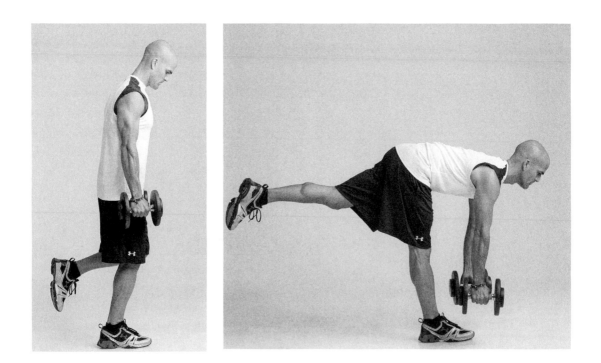

1. Begin with one foot flat on the ground, back straight, and abdominals contracted. Hold the dumbbells with your palms facing your body.

2. Slowly bend forward and lower the dumbbells toward your front foot, pushing your glutes back as you lift the other leg back and up.

3. Once you reach midshin level, flex your hamstring and push your hips forward to bring your body back to the start position.

4. Switch sides. Repeat 10 times with each leg.

>>tips:

Emphasize the hamstrings of the front leg; the rear leg is only used for balance. Keep your back straight and abdominals contracted.

exercise 3

ROMANIAN SPLIT SQUAT

Joints Engaged: Ⓢ Ⓗ Ⓚ

Muscles Worked: Primary–Quadriceps, Hamstrings; Secondary–Core, Shoulders

This is part lunge, part squat, and a complete leg builder.

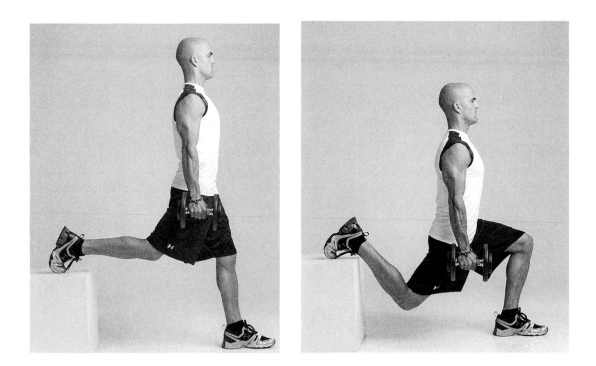

1. Begin with your back foot on an elevated surface; leg should be loose, with toes pointing down.

2. Squat down with your front leg until your thigh is almost parallel to the floor.

3. Push your body back to the start position using only the front leg.

4. Repeat 10 times, building up to 15.

5. Switch sides and repeat.

>>tips:

Make sure your front foot is positioned far enough in front of you so that your knee is in line with your heel when you squat down. Keep your back straight and your abdominals contracted.

BOSU-RESISTANCE PUSH-UP

Joints Engaged: Ⓢ Ⓔ Ⓗ Ⓚ

Muscles Worked: Primary—Chest; Secondary—Triceps, Shoulders, Core

A push-up is not a push-up. This variation places extra emphasis on core strength, stability, and balance.

1. Begin with your palms facing down on an upside-down bosu ball; position a resistance ball behind you.

2. Lift your feet onto the resistance ball while balancing your body on the bosu. Your body should be straight and toes pointed down.

3. When you are stable, do a classic push-up: Bend at the elbows and drop your upper body toward the bosu ball. Your feet remain up on the resistance ball.

4. Push yourself back up and repeat.

5. Repeat 10 times, building up to 20 reps.

>>tips:

Keep your body in a straight line
and your abdominals contracted.

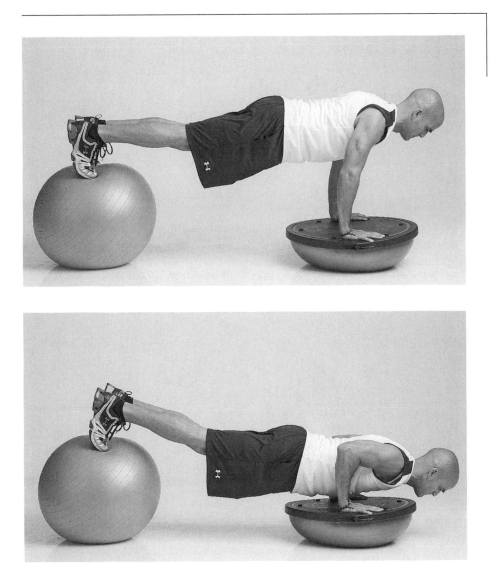

exercise 5

TOWEL DRAG

Joints Engaged: Ⓢ Ⓔ Ⓗ Ⓚ

Muscles Worked: Primary–Chest, Triceps; Secondary–Shoulders, Abdominals, Hip Flexors, Lower Back

This is also great on a carpeted surface with socks on your feet.

1. Begin with your legs straight, feet pointed down on the towel, your body extended; your palms should be facing down, shoulder width apart.

2. Drop down into a classic push-up position, elbows bent and close to your body.

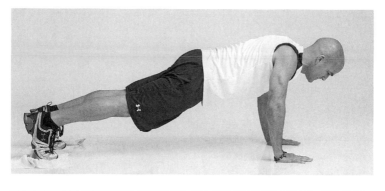

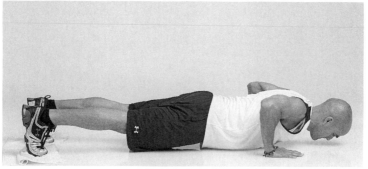

3. As you push yourself back up, slide your feet forward using the towel, as close to your body as possible. Your arms should be straight.

4. Slide your legs back to starting position, and repeat, beginning always with a push-up.

5. Repeat 10 times, working up to 20 reps.

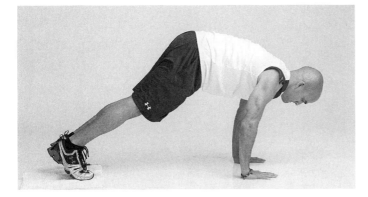

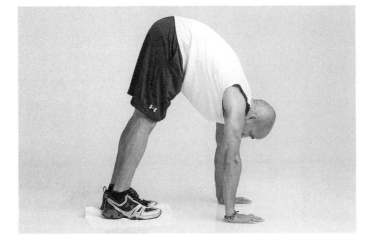

>>tips:

Try to make the move
one complete motion
from beginning to end.

exercise

6

L PULL-UPS

Joints Engaged: Ⓢ Ⓔ Ⓗ Ⓚ

Muscles Worked: Primary—Back, Core; Secondary—Biceps, Shoulders

This move builds incredible core strength.

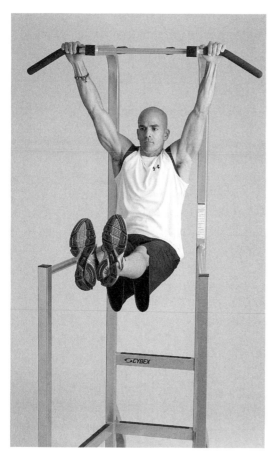

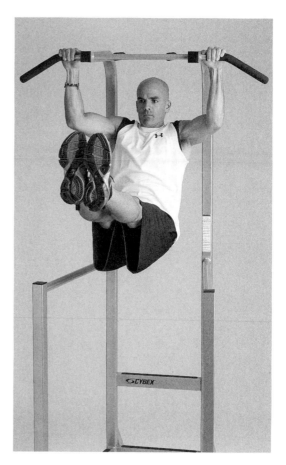

1. Begin in a classic pull-up position with your grip slightly wider than shoulder width. Your legs should be straight out in a 90-degree angle.

2. Pull up as far as you can, then return to starting position.

3. Repeat 10 times, building up to 20 reps.

>>**tips:**

Keep your knees locked, back straight, and do not swing.

exercise 7

SINGLE-LEG DUMBBELL CURL

Joints Engaged: E H K

Muscles Worked: Primary–Biceps; Secondary–Core, Shoulders, Legs

This twist on the classic curl develops balance, stability, and core strength.

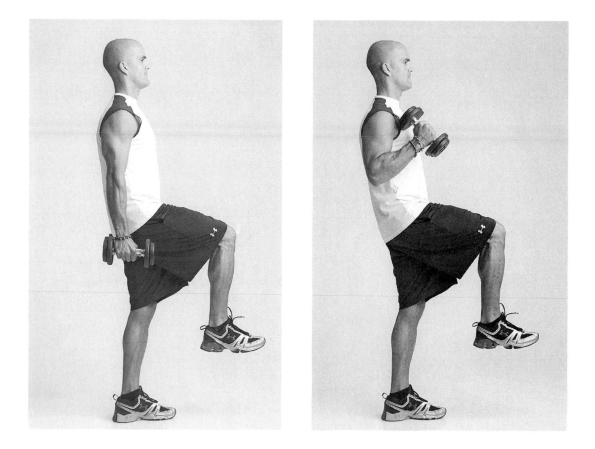

1. Begin with weight at either side of your body, palms facing in.

2. Balance your body on one leg as you lift the other in front of you.

3. Curl the dumbbells up and return to start position.

4. Repeat 10 times, building up to 15 reps.

5. Switch legs and repeat.

>>tips:
Keep your back straight and your abdominals contracted.

exercise

8

PARALLEL DIPS

Joints Engaged: 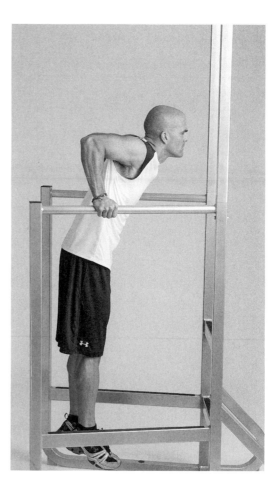 **S** **E**

Muscles Worked: Primary–Triceps; Secondary–Chest, Shoulders

A very simple move that yields incredible results.

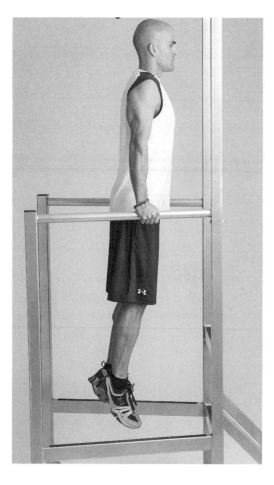

1. Place your hands on the parallel bars with arms straight and palms facing in. Your body should be lifted, weight on your arms.

2. Slowly lower yourself until your upper arms are parallel to the ground.

3. Slowly lift back up.

4. Repeat 10 times, building up to 20 reps.

>>tips:

Keep your back straight and your chest up.

SUSPENDED RESISTANCE-BALL SIT-UP

Joints Engaged: (H) (K)

Muscles Worked: Primary—Abdominals; Secondary—Hip Flexors, Lower Back

Not just a great abdominal move but also great for balance and stability.

1. Begin by sitting firmly on the resistance ball.

2. Lean back and hook your feet to something stable that isn't going to move.

3. Lower your upper body back until your body is a straight line parallel to the floor.

4. Rise back up to starting position.

5. Repeat 10 times, building up to 20 reps.

>>tips:

Think slow and controlled movements for maximum results.

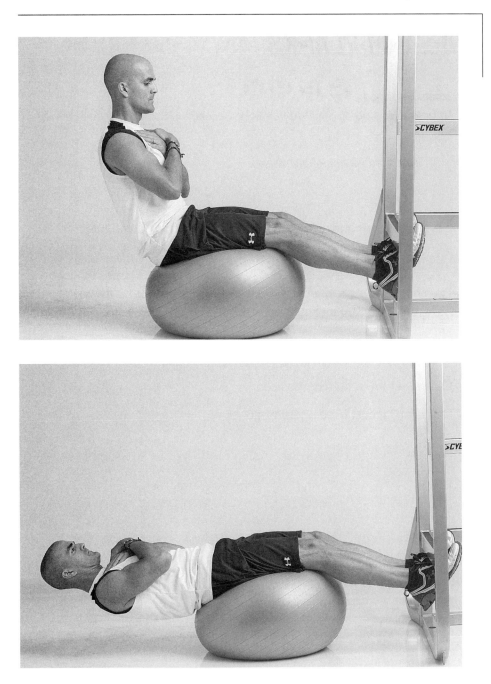

exercise
10

FOREARM PLANKS

Joints Engaged: Ⓢ Ⓔ Ⓗ Ⓚ

Muscles Worked: Primary–Abdominals; Secondary–Shoulders, Lower Back, Hip Flexors

Advanced version of the plank.

1. Start with your hands clasped together, elbows bent, and forearms leaning on a resistance ball. Your body should be in a straight line, legs extended, and toes pointing toward the floor.

2. You should now be in a classic plank position, except on the resistance ball. Your lower arms should be at a 90-degree angle from your upper arms.

3. Pull your elbows into your abdomen.

4. Quickly return to starting position.

5. Repeat 10 times, building up to 20 reps.

>>tips:

Your arms are the only body part that should move. Keep your back straight and your abdominals contracted.

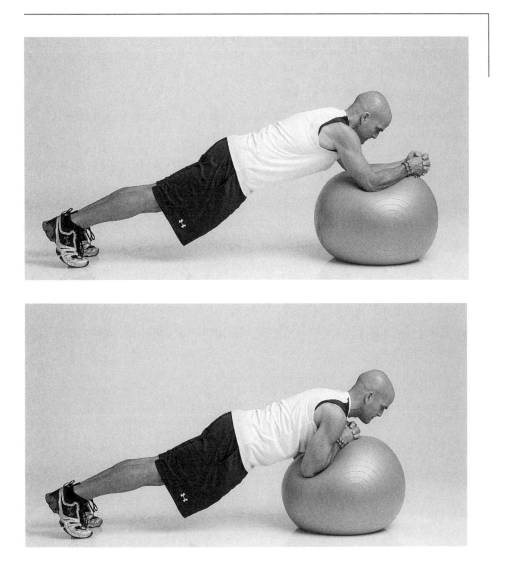

BARBELL OBLIQUE TWIST

Joints Engaged: Ⓢ Ⓗ Ⓚ

Muscles Worked: Primary–Obliques; Secondary–Shoulders, Triceps, Lower Back

This move can also be performed with dumbbells, a medicine ball, or even with no weight.

1. Starting position: You are lying down, back on the floor. Hold a barbell above your chest in a slightly wider grip than your shoulders. Palms should be facing out. Legs should be up at a 90-degree angle from your upper body. Knees should be locked.

2. Slowly lower your legs to one side of your body without moving your upper body.

3. Return to start position and repeat to opposite side.

4. Repeat 10 times on each side, building up to 20 reps.

>>tips:

Do not just drop your legs to the sides; the movement should be slow and controlled.

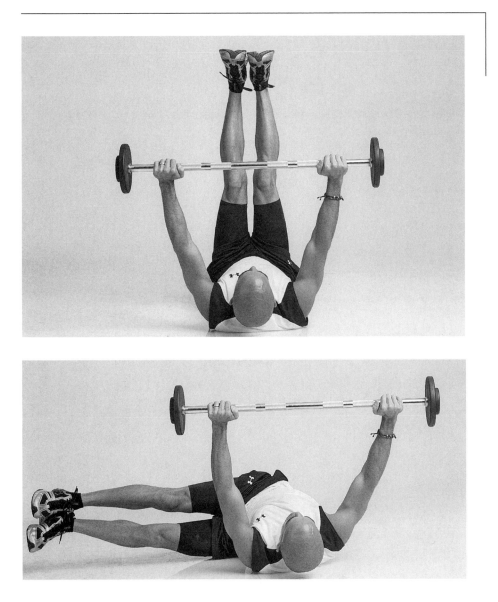

FIGURE 8S

Joints Engaged: Ⓢ Ⓔ Ⓗ Ⓚ

Muscles Worked: Primary—Obliques; Secondary—Hip Flexors, Lower Back, Shoulders, Biceps

This move requires some coordination but is extremely effective.

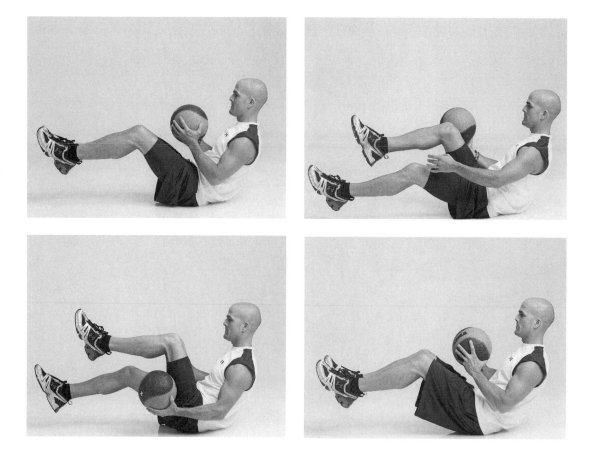

1. Begin in a seated position, buttocks on the floor. Your feet should be in front of you with your knees bent; your heels should be off the ground. Hold a medicine ball in both hands near your chest.

2. Raise one leg and pass the medicine ball between your legs (always pass through the middle).

3. Repeat with the other leg.

4. Repeat entire exercise 10 times, building up to 20 reps.

>>tips:

Imagine you are pedaling a bicycle: One knee goes up while the other goes down.

exercise
13

SINGLE-LEG PLANK

Joints Engaged: Ⓢ Ⓔ Ⓗ Ⓚ

Muscles Worked: Primary–Abdominals; Secondary–Lower Back, Hip Flexors, Shoulders, Triceps

The plank position is used extensively in all types of exercise, including Pilates and yoga.

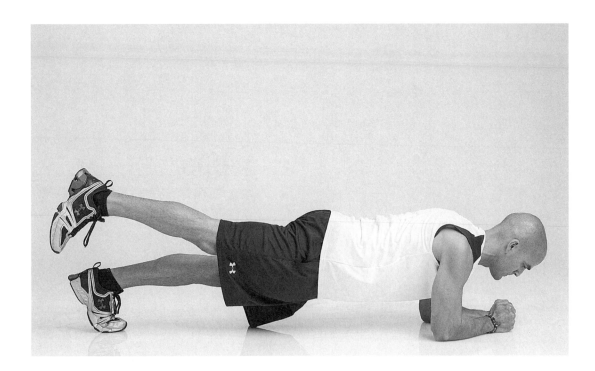

1. Begin with your forearms firmly on the floor, your feet shoulder width apart.

2. Lift one leg in the air and hold this isometric contraction (muscle length remains the same, although it is contracted) for 30 seconds.

3. Lower the leg.

4. Switch sides.

>>tips:

For an extra challenge, try straightening your arms and supporting your body with your palms instead of your forearms.

WARRIOR WORKOUT Option #2

Even warriors get bored. To vary an extremely challenging workout, try this!

DUMBBELL FRONT SQUAT

Joints Engaged: Ⓢ Ⓔ Ⓗ Ⓚ

Muscles Worked: Primary—Quadriceps; Secondary—Hamstrings, Glutes, Shoulders, Biceps, Triceps, Chest, Core

Unlike the traditional squat, which places the resistance (weight) behind the neck, this option places the resistance in front. It also places extra resistance on the upper body, adding shoulder, arm, and core work.

1. Begin with your feet shoulder width apart and one dumbbell between your hands at chin height.

2. Squat down, hips back, with your back straight and chest up until your elbows touch your knees.

3. Squeeze your legs and glutes, and return to start position.

4. Repeat 10 times, building up to 15 reps.

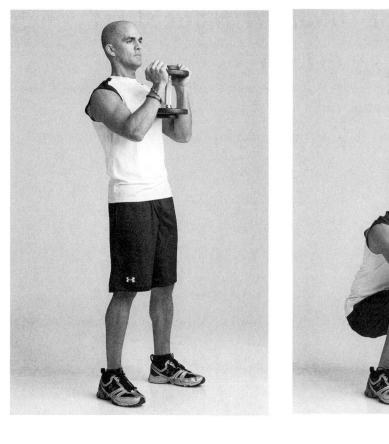

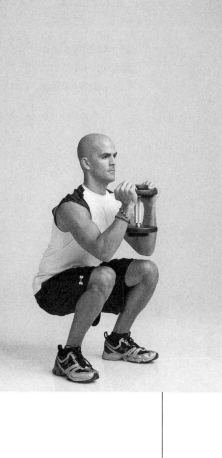

>>tips:

Keep your back straight and your
abdominals contracted.

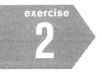

exercise 2

REVERSE LUNGE WITH CHEST FLY

Joints Engaged: Ⓢ Ⓔ Ⓗ Ⓚ

Muscles Worked: Primary—Quadriceps, Chest; Secondary—Hamstrings, Glutes, Biceps, Shoulders, Core

Another variation on a lunge, this time paired with an upper-body move.

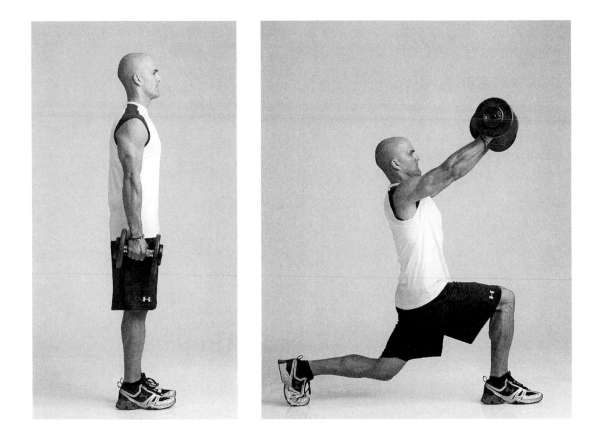

1. Begin in a standing position with your feet shoulder width apart and dumbbells at your sides, palms facing the body.

2. Step back into a reverse lunge with one foot and simultaneously press both dumbbells to arm's length in front of you. End with palms up.

3. Return to start position.

4. Switch sides. Repeat 10 times with each leg, for a total of 20 reps.

>>**tips:**

The knee of the forward leg should line up over the heel.

EXPLODING PUSH-UPS

Joints Engaged: Ⓢ Ⓔ Ⓗ Ⓚ

Muscles Worked: Primary–Chest; Secondary–Triceps, Shoulders, Core

Another challenging variation of the classic push-up.

1. Begin in a classic push-up position, but add a medicine ball under one hand.

2. Perform one push-up with the medicine ball under the hand.

3. As you return to start position, roll the medicine ball to the other hand and repeat the push-up. Continue to perform push-ups, alternating the ball from left hand to right.

4. Repeat 10 times with each hand, for a total of 20 reps.

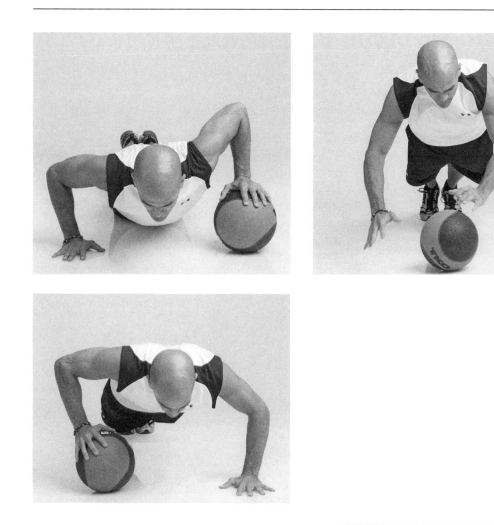

>>**tips:**

For real explosive results, try switching hands on the ball while still in the air! Keep your back straight.

RESISTANCE-BALL SINGLE-ARM PRESS

Joints Engaged: Ⓢ Ⓔ Ⓗ Ⓚ

Muscles Worked: Primary—Chest, Core; Secondary—Shoulders, Triceps

This chest press delivers a serious core workout.

1. Begin with your upper back on the resistance ball, elbows bent, and one dumbbell grasped in one hand.

2. Contract your core (pull in your abdominals) to stabilize your body, then extend the dumbbell straight up until the arm reaches a locked position.

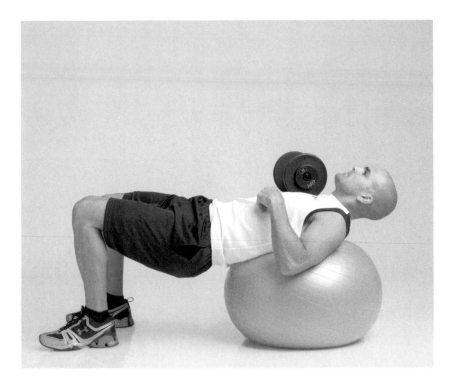

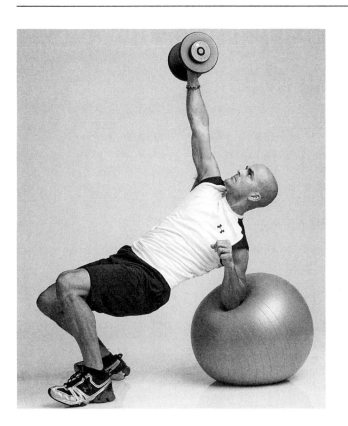

3. At the same time, quickly shift your body weight onto the opposite elbow and push the dumbbell even farther into the air.

4. Return to start position.

5. Repeat 10 times, building up to 15 reps.

6. Switch sides.

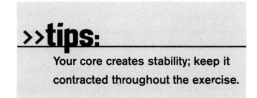

>>tips:

Your core creates stability; keep it contracted throughout the exercise.

SINGLE-LEG DUMBBELL ROW

Joints Engaged: Ⓢ Ⓔ Ⓗ Ⓚ

Muscles Worked: Primary–Back; Secondary–Biceps, Glutes, Shoulders, Core

All the obvious benefits and also a great way to work the proprioception (sense of orientation) of the ankle.

1. Begin with feet together and a dumbbell in each hand.

2. Lean forward and balance on one leg. Your arms should be hanging perpendicular to the floor.

3. Pull the dumbbells up and slightly back until they reach your lower chest.

4. Controlling the weight, slowly return to starting position in one smooth motion.

5. Repeat 10 times, building up to 15 reps.

>>tips:

Keep your back straight, core contracted, and weight-bearing knee slightly bent.

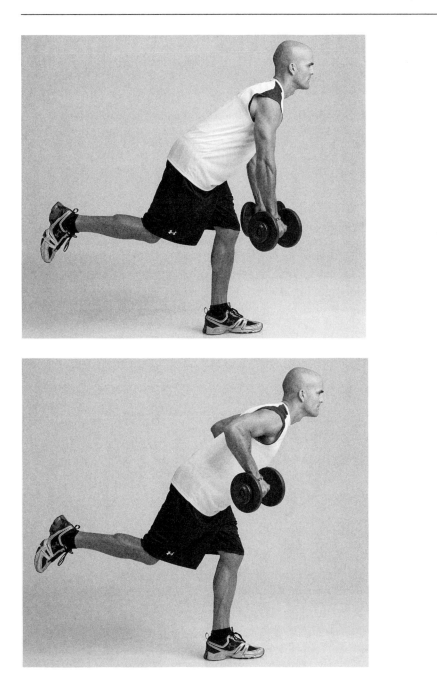

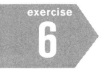

exercise 6

INCLINE BICEPS CURLS

Joints Engaged: Ⓢ Ⓔ Ⓗ Ⓚ

Muscles Worked: Primary–Biceps; Secondary–Shoulders, Core, Forearms

This is a great way to isolate the biceps and maintain a still upper body during the curl.

1. Position yourself on an incline bench, knees bent and suspended in the air. Grasp a dumbbell in each hand, palms facing in.

2. Bring the dumbbells up to your chest in a curling motion, bending at the elbows. Simultaneously turn the dumbbells so the palms are up at the top of the motion.

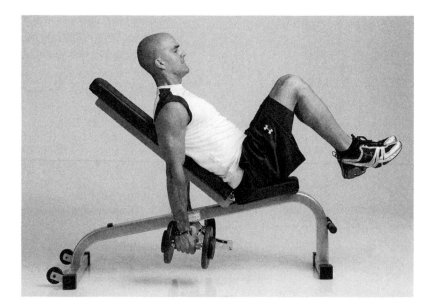

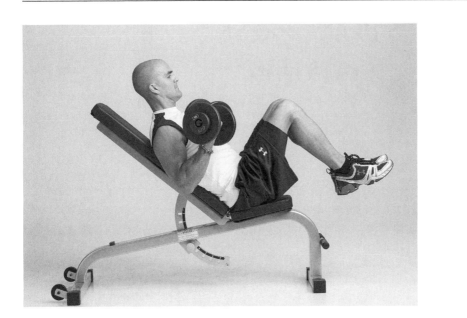

3. Return to starting position.

4. Repeat 10 times, building up to 15 reps.

>>tips:

Control the movement both ways: on the way up and on the way down.

exercise 7

TRICEPS PLANK PRESS

Joints Engaged: Ⓢ Ⓔ Ⓗ Ⓚ

Muscles Worked: Primary–Triceps; Secondary–Shoulders, Core

This builds unbelievable arm strength using only your body weight.

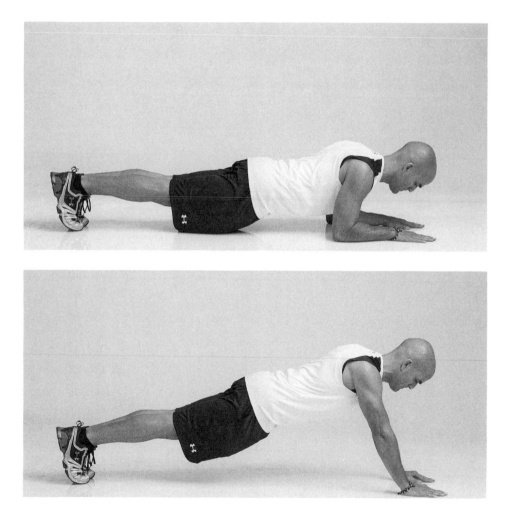

1. Begin in a classic push-up position with your hands placed slightly farther forward of your shoulders. Drop down into a plank position with elbows back.

2. Using your triceps, push yourself up, straightening your elbows; your shoulders should be slightly back.

3. Use your triceps to control your body weight as you bring your elbows back to the floor.

4. Repeat 10 times, building up to 15 reps.

>>**tips:**

Keep the elbows back throughout the movement. Maintain a straight line down the body.

exercise

8

DUMBBELL SHOULDER SNATCH

Joints Engaged: Ⓢ Ⓔ

Muscles Worked: Primary–Shoulders; Secondary–Core

Here is a twist on the snatch that athletes have been using for years.

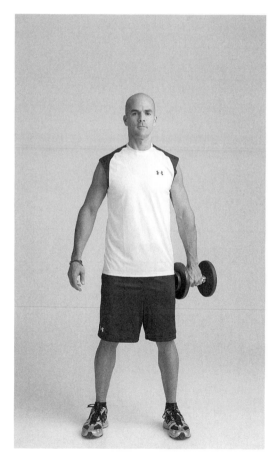

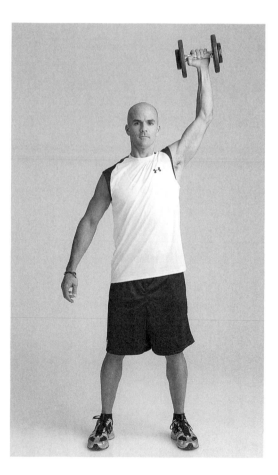

1. Starting position: standing, shoulders back, abs in. Grab a dumbbell in one hand, palm down.

2. Pull in your abdominals and, in one quick movement, "snatch" (a fast raising of the arm) the dumbbell into the air, arm extended.

3. Control the weight as you lower your arm to starting position.

4. Switch sides. Repeat 10 times with each arm, for a total of 15 reps.

>>tips:

This is an explosive movement used to develop speed and power. The "snatch" should be performed quickly, the return to starting position slowly..

exercise 9

HANGING KNEE RAISES

Joints Engaged: Ⓢ Ⓔ Ⓗ Ⓚ

Muscles Worked: Primary–Abdominals; Secondary–Biceps, Back, Hip Flexors

One of my personal favorites.

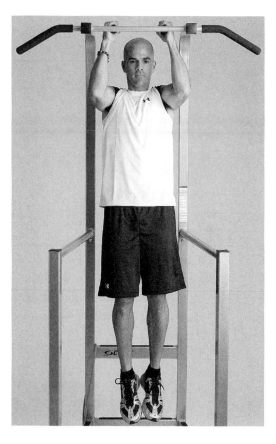

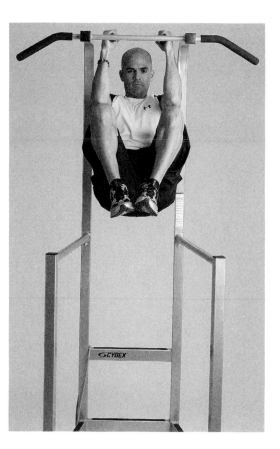

1. Begin hanging from a pull-up bar with a close grip, palms up. Maintain a 90-degree angle at the elbow joint.

2. Tuck your knees up into your chest.

3. Return to starting position.

4. Repeat 10 times, building up to 20 reps.

>>tips:

Try to touch your knees to your elbows with every repetition.

REACH AND TOUCH

Joints Engaged: Ⓢ Ⓔ Ⓗ Ⓚ

Muscles Worked: Primary—Abdominals, Hip Flexors; Secondary—Inner Thighs, Serratus Anterior (the muscles under the arm at the top of the rib cage), Biceps, Shoulders

This move places resistance on both the abdominals and hip flexors for an intense core workout.

1. Lie down on your back, body extended, with a medicine ball between your hands and a resistance ball held between your ankles. Hold both balls a few inches off the floor.

2. Pull in your abdominals as you lift both balls simultaneously toward each other.

3. Try to touch the two over the hips.

>>tips:

Keep arms and legs as straight as possible for maximum resistance.

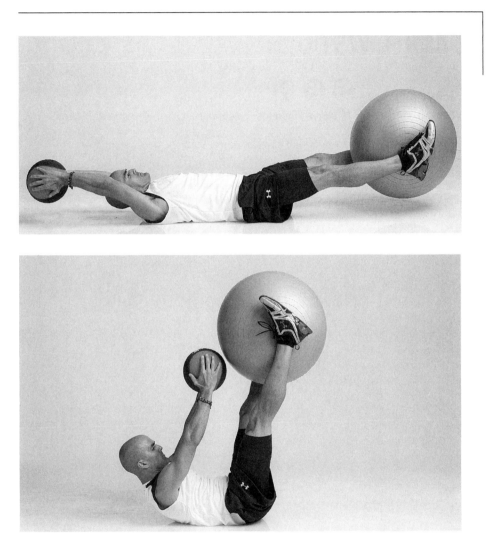

exercise
11

PLANK TWIST

Joints Engaged: Ⓢ Ⓔ Ⓗ

Muscles Worked: Primary–Obliques; Secondary–Core, Shoulders, Triceps

One move, three benefits: core strength, stability, and balance.

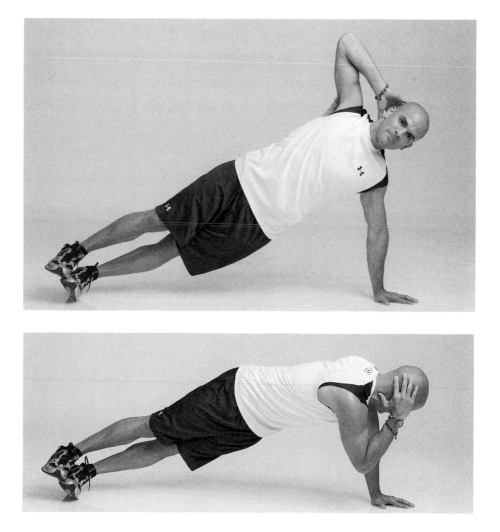

1. Begin on your side with your feet together, one on top of the other.

2. Place one arm on the floor, hand flat, arm extended, elbow locked. This arm will be holding your body weight.

3. Bend your free hand at the elbow and place it behind your head.

4. Reach with the elbow in a twisting motion toward the midpoint of the arm holding up your weight.

5. Return to start position.

6. Repeat 10 times, building up to 20 reps.

>>**tips:**

Do not drop your hips.

INCLINE BENCH REVERSE CRUNCH

Joints Engaged: Ⓢ Ⓔ Ⓗ Ⓚ

Muscles Worked: Primary–Abdominals, Hip Flexors; Secondary–Biceps, Serratus Anterior

This reverse crunch uses gravity as resistance.

1. Lie down on an incline bench with your hands behind your head holding on to the top edge of the bench.

2. Bend your knees and bring them up into the air, feet off the ground.

3. Pull up your knees and tuck them into your upper body.

4. Return to starting position.

5. Repeat 10 times, building up to 20 reps.

>>tips:

Try to touch your elbows with your knees with each repetition.

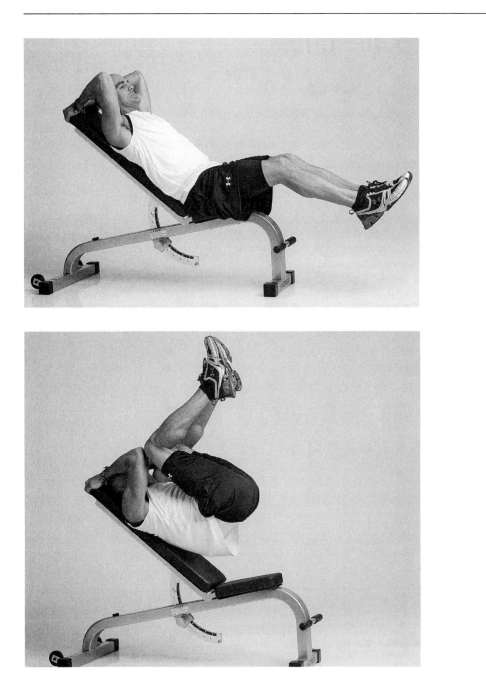

RESISTANCE CHOP

Joints Engaged: S E

Muscles Worked: Primary–Core; Secondary–Triceps, Shoulders

This can be performed with a cable pulley or resistance band.

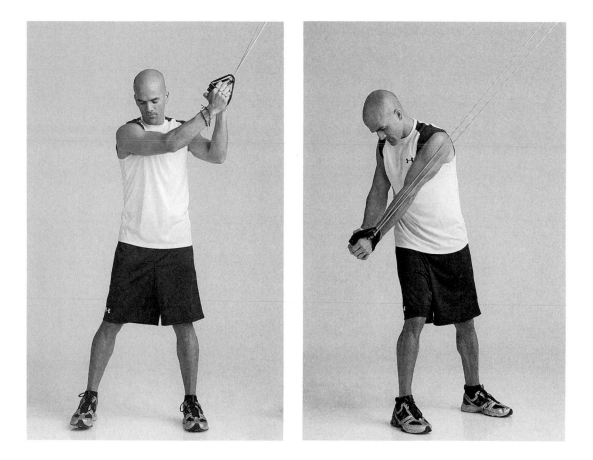

1. Begin with an overlapping grip on the handle of the cable pulley/ resistance band. Stand tall with a contracted core. The rope/band should be aligned with the top of your shoulder.

2. Pull the cable/band in a chopping motion across your body, ending at the opposite hip.

3. Return to starting position.

4. Repeat 10 times, building up to 15 reps.

>>tips:

Keep your core stable and engaged throughout this movement.

TRY THIS!

I love to challenge myself, and, if you're up for it, I think you might enjoy these four extra power exercises, too. Add these to any workout or try them alone.

exercise 1

MEDICINE BALL PISTOL SQUAT

Joints Engaged: Ⓢ Ⓔ Ⓗ Ⓚ
Muscles Worked: Total Body

This can also be performed on a bosu ball.

1. Begin with your feet together, a medicine ball held at chest height.

2. Lift one leg forward with knee locked and start to squat down with the opposite leg.

3. Squat all the way down until your buttock touches your heel—the other leg still straight out.

4. Return to starting position and repeat 10 times, building up to 15 reps.

5. Switch sides.

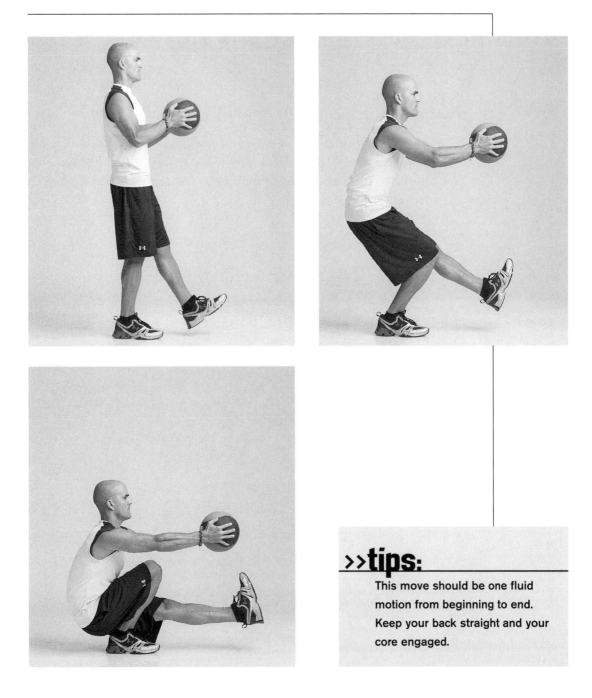

>>**tips:**

This move should be one fluid motion from beginning to end. Keep your back straight and your core engaged.

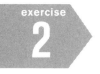

exercise
2

DUMBBELL JUMP-THROUGH

Joints Engaged: **S** **E** **H** **K**
Muscles Worked: Total Body

This exercise is quite advanced and requires balance when you do it with a pair of dumbbells. For the first few times, I suggest you try it with a pair of blocks (or some other steady object) instead of dumbbells to make sure you get it right.

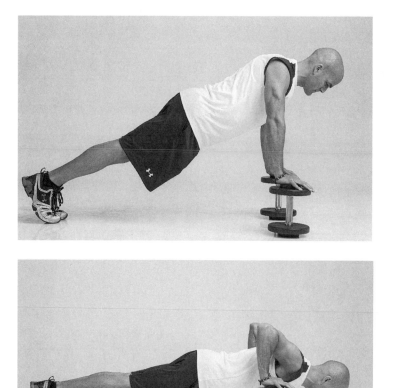

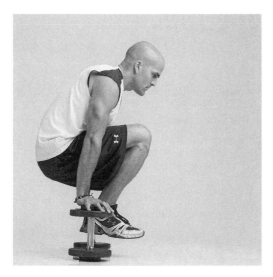
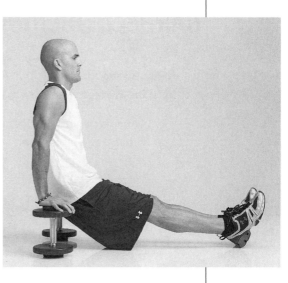

1. Begin in a push-up position with your hands on blocks (or dumbbells standing up on their ends). *If you're using dumbbells, be very careful— they can tip over!*

2. Perform a push-up. As you return to start position, tuck your knees and jump through your arms, then land in position for a reverse dip.

3. Perform a reverse dip and jump back through the arms, back to push-up position.

4. Repeat 10 times, building up to 20 reps.

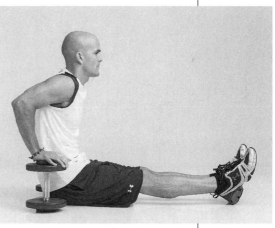

>>tips:

Stay light on your feet with your weight over your hands for easy jump-throughs.

exercise 3

BARBELL OBLIQUE TOE TOUCH

Joints Engaged: Ⓢ Ⓔ Ⓗ Ⓚ

Muscles Worked: Primary–Core; Secondary–Shoulders, Hamstrings

This exercise requires flexibility and core strength. Begin slowly and stop if you feel any discomfort.

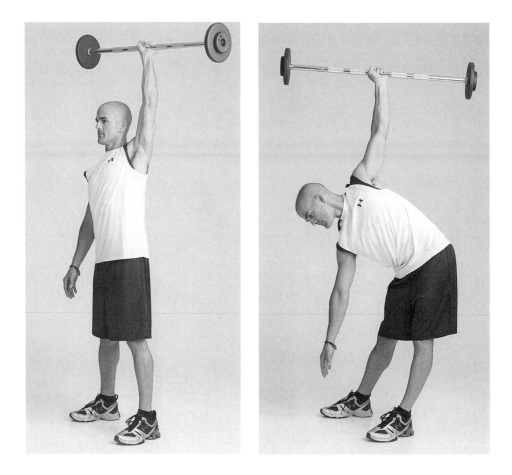

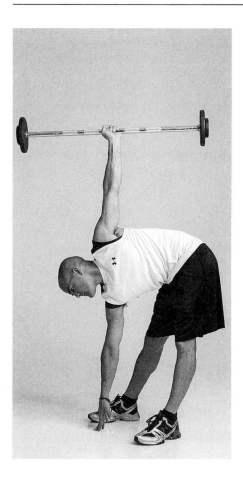

1. Begin in a standing position with your feet shoulder width apart. Hold a barbell overhead with one arm.

2. Slowly drop your chest with a straight back and reach for the floor in front of you—all the while keeping the barbell straight up in the air with the opposite hand. (At the bottom of the move, your arms should be stretched out in both extremes.)

3. Slowly rise back up.

4. Repeat 10 times, building up to 15 reps.

5. Switch sides.

>>tips:

Try the movement first without any weight. Once you have the motion down, repeat with a dumbbell. Once you're comfortable with a dumbbell, you can progress to the barbell.

exercise

4

MEDICINE BALL SIT-UP & STAND

Joints Engaged: Ⓢ Ⓔ Ⓗ Ⓚ

Muscles Worked: Primary–Abdominals; Secondary–Quadriceps, Shoulders, Core

This exercise takes the sit-up to a whole new level (literally!). Try it.

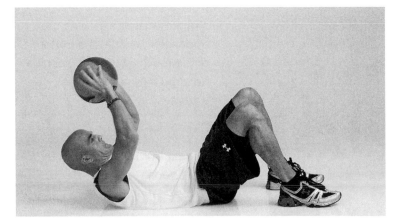

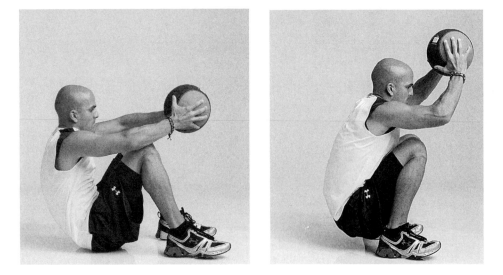

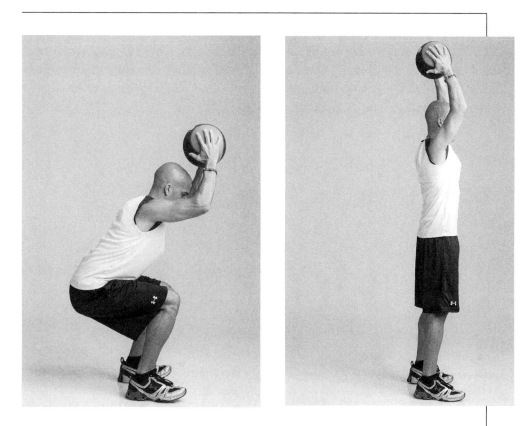

1. Begin on the floor on your back, knees bent.

2. Holding a medicine ball with two hands over your head, quickly sit up, leading with the medicine ball in front of you.

3. Using your abs and your quads, pull yourself up into a standing position. The medicine ball should be held out in front as a counterweight to help you get to the standing position. Once you're in standing position, you should hold the ball straight overhead with arms fully extended.

4. Slowly move back down and roll yourself out into starting position.

5. Repeat 10 times, building up to 20 reps.

>>tips:

Move quickly and use your body's momentum to stand.

CONCLUSION

These Power Moves are just a sampling of what you can do with the four motions (joints). I encourage you to feel free to mix up the exercises and create your own routines using the exercises you enjoy most. After all, if you don't enjoy exercising, chances are you won't remain consistent—and when it comes to health, fitness, and total wellness, **Consistency Is Key!!!**

POWER STRETCHING

Importance of Stretching

"Why should I stretch?"

"I don't have time to stretch!"

I've heard it all. But I can't stress enough the importance of stretching. Simply put, stretching makes you more flexible, and flexibility is a huge factor in your overall health and fitness.

Stretching also . . .

- Improves Range of Motion
- Improves Circulation
- Relieves Stress
- Prevents Injury
- Improves Posture
- Improves Coordination

We are born with an incredible range of motion (think of babies sucking on their toes), but as we get older most of us don't bother to work to maintain this range of motion—and as a result, it decreases. But by stretching, we can increase our range of motion, and in turn reduce the risk of injury.

Here are a few simple stretches to start with. Remember, don't overstretch. Stretching too far or too vigorously can be worse for you than not stretching at all. So start slow and be patient. It's probably been a while since you stretched, so don't expect to be like Gumby by tomorrow!

Some Tips to Remember

1. Warm up first: Stretching muscles when they're cold can actually increase your risk of injury. I prefer to stretch after my workouts because the muscles are warm deep at the core. But some people prefer to stretch beforehand. If you stretch before your workout, make sure to warm up for at least 10 minutes before stretching.

2. Target major muscle groups: Focus on your quads, hamstrings, lower back, chest, shoulders, and hips. Also make sure to stretch any muscles that you routinely use at work or play.

3. Hold your stretches initially for 10 seconds, and work your way up to 30–45 seconds.

4. Don't hold your breath: Relax and breathe naturally through the stretch-and-hold sequence.

5. Pain-free: It's normal for really tight muscles to feel uncomfortable to stretch, but it shouldn't ever feel painful. If you begin to feel pain, you've gone too far. Release the stretch to the point where you are pain-free and hold it there.

6. Don't bounce: Bouncing can cause injury (microtears) to the muscle. I prefer "static stretching" (holding a position), where you stretch to the farthest point and hold the stretch.

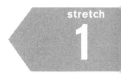

HAMSTRINGS STRETCH

Stretches: Hamstrings, Lower Back

Tightness in the hamstrings will place increased stress on the lower back and often aggravate—or even cause—some of the conditions that result in sciatica.

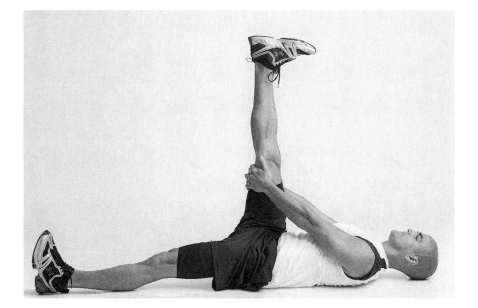

Lie on your back, supporting your thigh behind the knee with the hand or with a towel. Slowly straighten the knee until a stretch is felt in the back of the thigh, trying to get the bottom of the foot to face the ceiling, one leg at a time. Hold the stretch initially for 10 seconds, and gradually work up to 20–30 seconds. Switch legs and repeat.

KNEELING HIP FLEXOR/QUAD STRETCH

Stretches: Hip Flexor, Quads

I love this stretch because it gives the muscles in your quads an intensely deep stretch. Having tight quads can pull your patella (kneecap) out of line, which makes it a lot weaker, and also it will pull on your pelvis, which will affect your back. This is an important stretch to do after running and biking.

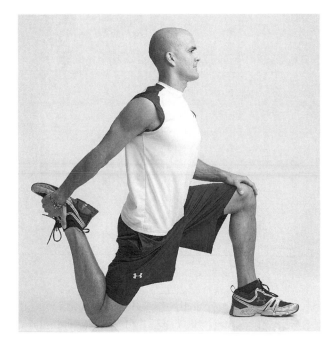

Fold up a towel and kneel down on it with your right knee. Now place your left foot on the ground in front of you and slowly drop your hips until you feel the stretch in the front of your right hip. Make sure your left knee is directly above your left ankle. Reach back, if you can, and grab your right ankle and slowly pull toward your buttocks. Hold the stretch initially for 10 seconds, and gradually work up to 20–30 seconds. Switch sides and repeat.

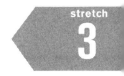

LYING TRUNK TWIST

Stretches: Lower Back

As many as 50 percent of all Americans report some type of back pain every year. Back pain causes not only a physical strain but also a financial one because of missed workdays, loss of productivity, and medical bills. Stretching makes a huge difference.

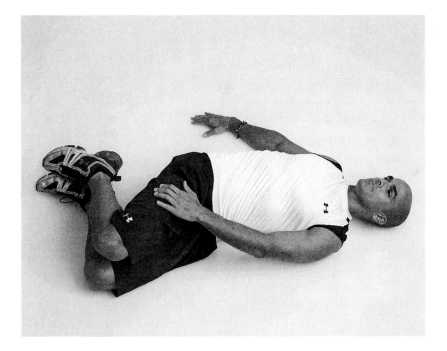

Lie flat on your back with both hands extended out to the sides. Bend your legs at the knees and drop both legs toward one arm, trying to keep your knees together, while allowing your lower body to twist around. You may also perform this stretch with legs straight. Hold the stretch initially for 10 seconds, and gradually work up to 20–30 seconds. Switch sides and repeat.

stretch

4

OVERHEAD LAT STRETCH

Stretches: Upper Back, Lats, Shoulders

This is great for loosening the muscles of the upper back and shoulders. For an additional stretch, once you are holding the stretch at the top, you may want to slowly reach to one side as you hold the pose. Simply tilt the upper body to the left and then to the right for an additional stretch.

Start by placing both hands together (you may interlace your fingers), then reach with the palms above your head as you slowly straighten your arms. Once you feel a slight stretch in the arms, shoulders, or upper back, hold the posi-tion. Hold the stretch initially for 10 seconds, and gradually work up to 20–30 seconds.

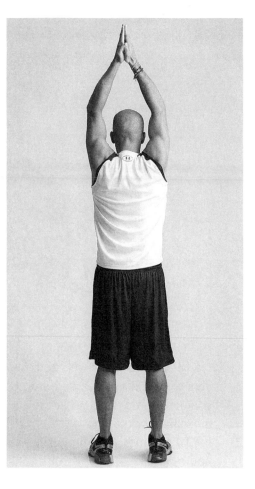

CHEST STRETCH

Stretches: Chest

The muscles of your upper body tend to become tight as you age, especially if you work behind a desk. Use this stretch not only to improve flexibility but also a few times a day to relax and improve circulation and energy level.

Stand up straight, with knees slightly bent. Place your feet shoulder width apart with your toes pointing forward. Place your arms behind your back and clasp hands together. Extend your arms behind your back, push your chest slightly forward, and hold this position. Hold the stretch initially for 10 seconds, and gradually work up to 20–30 seconds.

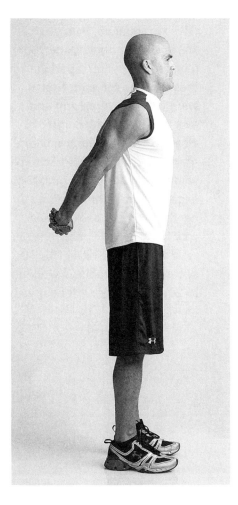

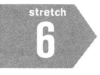

stretch
6

STANDING BICEPS STRETCH

Stretches: Biceps

The exercises you perform for beautifully toned arms can also rob you of your range of motion. So I recommend this stretch be performed after all arm workouts.

Stand up straight, with your knees slightly bent. Place your feet shoulder width apart with toes pointing forward. Reach forward with your right arm and lock it at the elbow once it's close to parallel with the floor (palm should be up). Reach up with the left hand and grab the fingers of the right hand and gently pull them back toward your body (mild hyperextension). Hold the stretch initially for 10 seconds, and gradually work up to 20–30 seconds. Repeat with the other arm.

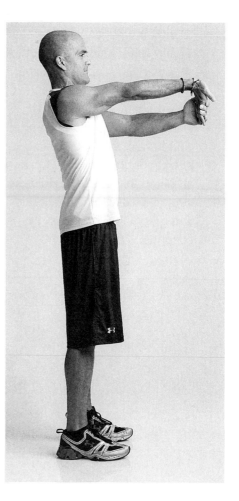

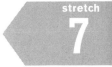

TRICEPS OVERHEAD

Stretches: Triceps

I love this one, especially after a long bike ride. This stretch will not only help increase the flexibility of your triceps but will also loosen your shoulders and upper back.

Stand up straight, with your knees slightly bent. Place your feet shoulder width apart with toes pointing forward. Place one arm overhead and bend at the elbow. Grab the elbow overhead with the other hand and hold. Hold the stretch initially for 10 seconds, and gradually work up to 20–30 seconds. Repeat with the opposite arm.

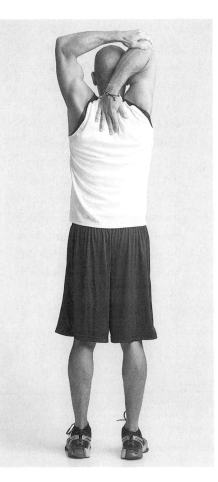

stretch

8

CROSS-BODY SHOULDER STRETCH

Stretches: Shoulders

Because the shoulder has the greatest range of motion of any joint in the body, it is also more likely to be injured or develop overuse injuries. Stretching the shoulder is a great way to preserve flexibility and range of motion. After all, the shoulder joint moves every time you move your arms, so even when you're not working out you're still stressing the joint.

Stand up straight, with your knees slightly bent. Place your feet shoulder width apart with toes pointing forward. Bend your right arm at the elbow joint, and extend the arm across your chest. Place your left hand on your right elbow to gently support the arm during the stretch. Hold the stretch initially for 10 seconds, and gradually work up to 20–30 seconds. Repeat with the opposite arm.

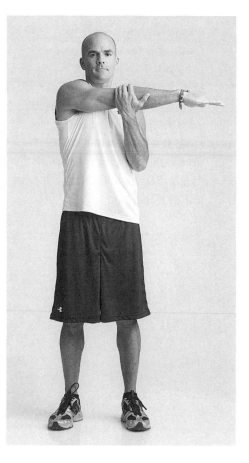

YOGA

Before we move on from stretching, I want to bring up a subject that I often get asked about: yoga. Yoga has gotten very popular in recent years, and for good reason. It has many restorative and rejuvenating properties. It:

1. Calms and soothes your mind
2. Massages your internal organs
3. Improves posture
4. Lubricates your joints
5. Tones muscle
6. Increases flexibility
7. Reconnects mind and body
8. Tones the core

For those who have never tried yoga and are quick to dismiss it, I always say, "Think of yoga as going in for a great stretch session and leaving with a whole lot more for free."

Power Eating

"It's not about dieting;
it's about changing
the way you think
about food."

People ask me all the time, "Marco, what diet do you recommend?"

But the truth is, I don't believe in diets.

Let me be clear: There's nothing wrong with—or shameful about—wanting to lose weight quickly. I've helped lots of people accomplish this kind of short-term goal. And with my Power Moves programs, and the Power Eating advice that I'm about to share with you, you will have all the tools you need to accomplish such a goal.

But you can also achieve so much more.

I'm talking *permanent* weight loss, and not feeling like you're starving or depriving yourself of all that is fun and carefree in life.

I'm talking about feeling good, and establishing healthy eating *habits* as opposed to rigid diets. Habits that come naturally and aren't forced.

It sounds too good to be true, I know. But it's actually very simple.

All it takes is changing the way you *think* about food.

I've seen lots of people fall victim to the same pattern. They want to lose weight quickly—say, five or ten pounds—in order to look good at a wedding or a beach vacation or some other event. So they go on a crash regimen of only juice or only cabbage or only this or that. And they succeed in achieving their goal. But what do you think happens then? What happens once they've lost the pounds and gotten their body looking how they want it to look?

The diet falls apart, of course. It falls apart because the person never changed the way they *think* about food and about their eating habits. So the minute they reach their goal, they return to their old behavior—and ultimately to their old body. Despite that initial motivation and that take-charge sprint, once the dieter reaches their goal, he or she almost always slows down. Maybe the diet lasts a few weeks, even a few months, but eventually those feelings of deprivation creep in and the bad eating habits return.

This is why I don't believe in diets. I'll say it again: Good health and permanent weight loss is not about dieting, it's about changing the way you *think* about food.

It's easy to do, and in this section I will show you how. You will look and feel great, and not just for an upcoming wedding, not just for the beach season—for life. But before we get into the nuts and bolts of how to change the way you think about eating, let's start by going over some general principles and some common pitfalls that occur when people are trying to lose weight—and how you can avoid these pitfalls.

We'll now turn to the examples of Elaine, John, Rhonda, and Diane, and see how the stories of these four individuals represent four important principles of weight loss for life. . . .

FOUR IMPORTANT PRINCIPLES OF WEIGHT LOSS FOR LIFE

PRINCIPLE #1: The key to permanent weight loss is to establish healthy eating *habits*, as opposed to strict diets that are all about deprivation.

Elaine and Her Deprivation Mentality

Elaine looked pretty good. She wanted to tone and strengthen her body, but she didn't look like she needed to lose weight.

But Elaine was adamant: She'd just lost ten pounds with a liquid diet and she wanted to lose ten more. There's nothing shameful about having a goal like this, but I could see that she was thinking about it the wrong way. She should have been focusing on a nutritious eating plan for both short-term and permanent weight loss, a plan that would have given her a blueprint for a happy and healthy life. Instead, it soon became clear that she believed the only way to a thinner body was through deprivation and even virtual starvation. Elaine hadn't exercised in a while, but she didn't have the energy for it either. (When you deprive or starve yourself, you have less energy, and so your drive and desire for exercise are diminished.)

She tried—and even forced herself—to exercise, but it was clear to me that exercise wasn't her biggest issue. Until she stopped depriving herself of food, there was no way she was going to be able to exercise. I tried to introduce her to my Power Eating plan for permanent weight loss and wellness—lots of nutritious foods, such as fruits, vegetables, whole grains, legumes, lean proteins, and healthy fats. But this approach just didn't make sense to her. It went against everything she always thought about dieting because it didn't involve depriving herself or starving. A diet that included fat? What kind of a diet was that?! A diet where you actually get to eat real food and not feel hungry all day? That will never work! That's how Elaine thought.

It took a while for her to come around but eventually she learned how to establish healthy eating habits and not deprive herself. Elaine managed to not just achieve her short-term goal of losing ten pounds but also to keep the weight off and be healthy and happy and not obsessed with dieting.

There's nothing wrong with having a short-term goal of wanting to lose a certain amount of weight in a certain amount of time, or of wanting to look good for a wedding or a vacation. It's helpful to set goals for yourself, and with my Power Moves programs and the Power Eating advice in this chapter, you will have all the tools you'll need to accomplish your goal.

But the long-term goal of permanent weight loss, and health and fitness for life, simply cannot be achieved if you don't put aside your preconceived notions and stop thinking about losing weight as "dieting" or depriving yourself.

I've seen it over and over again. If you try to diet in the sense of depriving yourself, what happens is you end up miserable, depressed, and so pent up that, like a dying man finally finding water in the desert, you'll overcompensate and gorge yourself.

Thinking about losing weight in terms of dieting-as-deprivation is sure to fail in the long run, because you will inevitably end up thinking about nothing but this deprivation. You'll lose sight of the real reason you were dieting (optimal health), and ironically you'll be so focused on the feelings of deprivation that it will be that much harder to achieve your short-term goals as well.

To summarize: You don't need to deprive yourself. You can learn to lead a healthy lifestyle that's also satisfying and pleasurable—and one that will make you look and feel great!

POWERtips >> WE ARE ALL born with the natural ability to listen to our internal hunger cues. Babies know when they are hungry and when they are full and when to stop eating. But as we get older we have a tendency to stop listening to these cues. We automatically just finish what's in front of us, as opposed to stopping when we're full. But with practice, we can go back to how we were as babies and learn to be in tune again with our natural hunger cues.

PRINCIPLE #2: Thinking about eating healthy and exercising isn't the same as actually eating healthy and exercising. I've heard so many people say, "This doesn't work for me, it's not in my genes, I work out and eat right and nothing . . ." Be careful not to fall into this trap. Be aware of your habits and behavior. What are you really eating, not just for breakfast, lunch, and dinner but also in between meals? And how much are you eating? Also, how much are you really exercising and how often?

John and His "Sluggish Metabolism"

John laughs about it now, but a few years ago he was convinced he couldn't lose weight. He had a high-powered job as a corporate lawyer and food was always something he ate either on the fly or over a business meeting. But he still tried to eat healthy—salad, salmon, and the like. He also had an elliptical trainer in his office and he'd use it when he got in to work in the morning, or when he was on the phone or had a few minutes to spare. Despite the cardio and what he thought was a relatively healthy diet, he still couldn't seem to lose weight.

Sounds reasonable, right? Here was a guy who maybe worked a little too hard at his job but who was really trying to have a healthy lifestyle. Well, the reality was that John was fifty pounds overweight—in spite of the salmon and the elliptical machine.

What was he doing wrong? John blamed it on a slow metabolism, but it had a lot more to do with the fact that he was just "going through the motions" of eating healthy. He was doing the same with his elliptical—just going through the motions, not working hard enough on the equipment, or with any consistency.

John decided to take action and began recording his food intake and exercise. To his surprise, his supposedly slow metabolism wasn't the culprit at all. Turns out that healthy salmon he was eating was covered in crème fraîche sauce. The salads were swimming in creamy dressing. In the same way that John was just going through the motions with his cardio, spending time on the elliptical but never coming close to breaking a sweat, he was also going through the motions with his supposedly healthy eating. He was eating stuff that's supposed to be good for you, but knowing deep down that he wasn't being genuine about it.

But once he started to record his calories, he began to realize the error of his ways and change his eating habits. These days, John has a genuinely healthy diet, one that doesn't just sound healthy but actually is healthy! And delicious!

POWERtips >> THE HUMAN BODY can easily consume 1,000 calories in just minutes. To burn that same number of calories would take over an hour of strenuous exercise. Don't use working out as an excuse to overeat.

When you're on a diet, you often say to yourself, "Okay, as long as I'm eating whatever the diet prescribes, eating lots of vegetables, fruit, fish, whole grains, and so on, I'm fulfilling my part of the bargain." You're following the dictates of the diet, but only in the most literal way. You're not following the logic *behind* the diet, so you're really just going through the motions.

Some, like John, eat the thing they know they're supposed to eat but drench it in unhealthy condiments or sauces. Others eat the healthy thing for their main meals but somehow forget about the random snacks, the muffin here, the piece of chocolate there—or they think it's okay to snack because they're working out. And others think it's all right for them to eat infinite quantities of a certain food if it's a food that their diet allows.

In all of these cases, the root problem is the same. The dieter is not seeing the forest for the trees. Subconsciously or not, he or she is just going through the motions of eating healthy without truly eating healthy. Think about it like this: Merely stepping on an elliptical or participating in a spinning class, in a lackluster way, won't make you fit, right? You have to put some energy into it. Well, it's the same with healthy eating. You have to do it like you mean it! But the good news is that once you start to see the great results that come from eating healthy, you'll genuinely be inspired to continue.

POWERtips >> NO MATTER HOW much money you make, if you spend more than you make you'll never have any money. Right? Well, the same goes with healthy eating and exercise. If you burn 1,000 calories a day through exercise but you overcompensate and eat an additional 2,000 calories a day, do you think you'll ever lose weight and be healthy?

PRINCIPLE #3: If you feel like you made a poor choice or you slipped up a bit, remind yourself it's not the end of the world. Don't use it as an excuse to lose control; learn from it and move forward.

Rhonda and the Chocolate Chip Cookie

You know that expression "I never met a cookie I didn't like"? Well, it's nowhere near as true as it is with Rhonda. She loved her cookies, and she could never have just one.

Knowing that cookies were a real trigger for her, she tried to stay away from them. Instead, she concentrated on eating healthy high-fiber, protein-rich foods. She also worked out four times a week. For a while, things were going great—she was looking good and feeling good.

But then one day she ate a cookie, and instead of just enjoying it and moving on, she figured "I blew it" and proceeded to chow down the whole bag. Because she'd veered ever so slightly off of her healthy eating habits, she decided she might as well fall all the way off.

This all-or-nothing way of thinking is very common. But have you ever met anyone who got fat from eating just one cookie? Of course not! Think about it as if it were a boxing match: You don't lose if you fall down—you lose if you *stay* down.

What I told Rhonda was to go ahead and have her one or two cookies, and enjoy it! And this advice worked. Once she understood the principle, she became more aware of her all-or-nothing behavior and was able to change it. Now when she has a craving for a treat, she indulges herself. But she only has a few, not the whole bag. Remember, the point is to change the way you *think* about food, to establish healthy eating habits—not to deprive yourself of something you love. And if you've really *earned* it, you should definitely go ahead and enjoy it. It's just like with work. If you work overtime for two weeks in a row in order to save some extra money to buy that purse you've been dreaming of, then you deserve it and you shouldn't feel bad.

There is a term that therapists use for certain clients: "catastrophic thinking." It's used to describe a person who thinks only in absolutes: He's either happy or he's sad; she's either perfect or she's the worst.

Of course, the reality is usually somewhere in the middle.

Catastrophic thinking is what happens when you go into all-or-nothing eating mode. By this I mean, for example, when you "blow" a diet by eating a bagel with cream cheese for breakfast, and so you figure you might as well not bother eating healthy for the whole rest of the day—and night. And then you wake up the next day and say, "Well, I blew yesterday, so I'll just start again on Monday" (which happens to be in three days!).

Before you know it you are gaining weight instead of losing it.

I'm sure you can see how illogical all of this is; one bagel does not spell doom. If you are going to eat a cookie, then you should enjoy it, savor it, really taste it. A treat is part of a healthy lifestyle. You can have an occasional treat—and in fact you should. When you change the way you think about food and establish healthy eating habits, you look at the bigger picture and you stop worrying about each little thing you eat.

PRINCIPLE #4: We are programmed from childhood to use food as an emotional crutch. By recognizing that emotional eating only compounds our problems we are able to break the cycle and move toward positive lifestyle changes.

Diane and the Comfort of Comfort Foods

Diane was what you would call an "emotional eater." She would bury her sorrows in food whenever she got bad news, such as when she was fired from her job as an account manager. Business had been down and she was laid off. A coworker offered to take her out for a drink, but Diane declined. She preferred to do her "drug of choice" alone at home. Diane's drug was food, the more refined carbs, the more sugar and salt, the better.

Out of work for a month, Diane had gained twenty pounds. She was feeling down on herself—mentally and physically—and she wasn't inspired to seek out new job prospects. The challenge was, as a first step, to help her learn how to transform her emotional eating habits into the kind of healthy eating habits that can turn your life around.

The phenomenon of "emotional eating" is easy to explain and its roots are obvious. From early childhood, the concept of food as a pain reliever is ingrained in us. As kids, when we felt sad we were offered sweets. When we got a bump on our head or scraped a knee, ice cream did the trick.

In other words, we are *programmed* to think this way. But the good news is we can break the cycle. All of us are capable of doing it. All it takes is recognizing these unhealthy patterns and changing the way you think about food. In the case of Diane, she made a conscious decision to wait ten minutes before reaching for that food, for that edible comfort. During those ten minutes she began to think rationally about the consequences of her actions. She thought about how eating that food would make her feel after the fact, and most important how it really wouldn't do anything to solve her original problem. She quickly realized that she was only making matters worse for herself and found other ways (positive ways) to cope with her emotions. Diane began an exercise program and used this time to come up with ways to get her life back on track, both personally and professionally.

POWERtips >> JUNK FOOD MAY taste good while you're eating it, but guilt and regret will soon follow. Why not make healthy choices that will taste great while making you feel and look your best?

FOOD IS THE MOST WIDELY ABUSED SUBSTANCE ON EARTH

Some people drink. Others turn to drugs. And many more turn to food when they are feeling bad.

It's understandable that we behave this way. It's been ingrained in us ever since we were kids that food will "turn that frown upside down." Think of the barber who gives the little boy a piece of gum to get him to stop squirming. Or the soccer coach who takes the team out for pizza to cheer them up after losing a game.

We're not kids anymore, but there's still that connection in our brain, so swift it's unconscious, that the best way to cope with something bad is to eat.

Here are some tips that help in dealing with emotional eating:

1. **When you feel the need to go to the fridge, stop and wait ten minutes.** If you still feel hungry, then go ahead—but chances are you'll make the healthy choice now that you've thought about it.
2. **Eat slowly,** resting your hand or putting down your utensils between every bite. Studies show that it takes twenty minutes after eating for your body to signal your brain that it's full. If you eat fast and furious, you won't give your body a chance to call it quits.

3. **Never eat standing up.** I've noticed that people who eat while hovering over their kitchen sink, for example, tend not to actually remember the food they ate. Whereas when you sit down at a table to a proper meal, there's a ritual to it—so you remember it.

4. **Never eat right out of the bag or box.** Put the cookies on a plate and the chips in a bowl. Emotional eaters often have a problem with "unconscious eating"—they reach into that package, grab a handful and take a bite, over and over again, and before they realize it they've finished the whole thing.

5. **Be aware of your emotional eating.** Recognize that eating junk food doesn't make your problems go away. In fact, it just gives you another problem, on top of the original problem. And, again, it might feel good for those thirty seconds while you're eating it, but when you establish healthy eating habits, the food tastes good and it feels good all day long.

6. **Buy what you need.** If you get into the habit of buying enough food for just a few days, you reduce the risk of bingeing.

POWERtips >> STAY AWAY FROM buying foods in bulk. When you buy a huge box or package of something, you're inclined to pour yourself a bigger serving. Instead, try to buy foods that are separated into individual packs and are designed for one serving at a time.

Although these four examples—Elaine, John, Rhonda, and Diane—were altered for the purpose of examples, their stories have been pieced together from real experiences and they represent four of the most important principles in establishing healthy eating habits and transforming your body for life.

YOU CAN LOSE WEIGHT

Calories are no mystery.

Diets are no mystery.

If you put in less than you expend, you will lose weight. Period.

It is in *your* power to lose weight and keep it off. How? By consciously choosing to eat more of the right foods and keeping up with your Power Moves exercise regimen.

Eating less.
Exercising more.

That's it. No secrets. No miracles. Just plain and simple truth.

It can't be said enough:
diets don't work.

I don't give my clients a diet. Instead, I educate them about food and help them make wise choices. Everyone is different and everyone has different triggers and traps. I believe in a healthy lifestyle that is created to fit the individual.

Before we go on to better, more powerful eating, I want you to answer the questions in the next section about your eating behavior. This will help you fashion your powerful eating plan so it will be successful for you.

> **POWERtips >>** WHY IS IT that when we're sick, we'll do anything to get ourselves feeling better—medicine, missing work, even surgery? But once we've recovered from the sickness, we don't devote the same energy to staying better. It's the same with eating healthy. We'll do anything to lose weight, but once we've lost it we don't work as hard to keep it off. When you change the way you *think* about food, you will change your perspective. You will learn how to focus on staying healthy for life.

RECOGNIZING YOUR EATING HABITS:
47 QUESTIONS

Losing weight is easy when it's on paper. You can look at, say, a two-week diet on your computer screen or in a book and think, "This looks easy. I can do this for two weeks. What's two weeks?" But of course we know that by day three, those two weeks seem like forever. That's because the diet is not tailored just for you. It doesn't take into account the way you like to eat, the foods you like to eat, or the times of the day you eat.

In order for a weight-loss plan to be successful, you need to think outside the box. It's not about "sticking" to a specific diet. No, it's about what works for you. It's all about behavior—and in order to change your behavior, you have to create your own individual program. Sure, there are foods we all need to stay away from, for weight loss and for good health. And, yes, the amount of food you eat can influence the number of pounds you lose. But there are ways to adapt a program to fit your lifestyle—to make it work outside the confines of a diet box.

The following questions will help you do just that. Your answers will reflect:

- the type of person you are: for example, a night owl or a morning person.
- your personal food triggers that you need to stay far, far away from.
- your eating routines: for example, do you usually eat while watching TV or do you dine out?
- your weight-loss behavior: for example, are you a yo-yo dieter or an unconscious eater?

Grab a piece of paper and a pen or pencil and begin. . . .

YOUR ROUTINES

1. Do you get hungry at night?
2. Are you a morning person?
3. Do you get the "munchies" at a certain time every day?
4. Do you work so hard that you sometimes forget to eat—and then feel famished?
5. Do you watch TV when you eat?
6. Do you always eat with your family or with friends?
7. Do you like to dine alone?
8. Do you eat a lot of frozen entrées? Do you think, Who has time to cook?
9. Do you love to cook?
10. Do you plan ahead, making weekday meals on Sundays?
11. Do you often eat standing up?
12. Is the first thing you do when you come home open the fridge?
13. Is there nothing in your refrigerator except some moldy cheese and a half-drunk bottle of wine?

How did you answer these? Jot down your responses and then move on to . . .

MY LIKES AND DISLIKES

14. Are you a junk-food junkie?
15. Do you try to eat organic as much as possible?
16. Are you a steak-and-potatoes person?
17. Do you love salad—but need dressing to make it edible?
18. Do you eat a lot of fish?
19. Do you like sweet foods?
20. Do you like salty foods?
21. Could you eat a pound of pasta if no one was looking?
22. When you're eating your favorite snack, do you go through an entire box or bag as if you're on autopilot?
23. Are you a chocoholic?
24. Do you only like to eat vegetables if they have some kind of sauce?
25. Do you love peanut butter—on just about everything?

How did you answer these? Write down your responses and then go to . . .

MY WEIGHT-LOSS BEHAVIOR

26. Can you never seem to take off those last five pounds?
27. Have you lost and gained the same twenty pounds all your life?
28. Do you hate measuring food when you're on a diet?
29. Do you record everything you eat?
30. Do you want to look great for an upcoming event or occasion?
31. Is your idea of looking thin to disguise yourself: to wear a sarong on the beach, and big long T-shirts when you're out and about? Or to never wear a shirt with a belt?
32. Are you more interested in building muscle than losing weight?
33. Do you want to lose at least thirty pounds?
34. Does your doctor say you have to lose weight for your health?
35. Do you just want to be able to maintain your current weight?

Again, jot down your responses and move on . . .

MY ACTIVITY LEVELS

36. Do you have a gym membership but don't use it very often?

37. Do you love to walk?

38. Do you usually use the stairs at work instead of the elevators?

39. Do you spend a lot of time on the couch in front of the TV?

40. Do you love taking naps?

41. Are you an indoor person?

42. Do you hate exercise even though you know it's good for you?

43. Are you intimidated by gyms? Do you feel unfamiliar with the equipment?

44. Do you feel comfortable using the weights at your gym by yourself, or do you need someone standing over your shoulder?

45. Do you go to the gym religiously? Would you consider yourself a regular?

46. As soon as the sun comes up, are you out there doing something?

47. Do you love exercise classes—the harder the better?

Jot down your responses from this section on your list.

Now look over the results from all four sections. These are your eating habits, your daily routines—what I call "the power of you."

There are no right answers or wrong answers. The idea is just to give you a chance to see who you are in an organized way. This is the first step in helping you establish healthy eating habits that are personalized and just right for you. For example, if you answered yes to the question about liking to cook, perhaps you should think about investing in a healthy cookbook. Or if you answered yes to the question about dining out a lot, you could look for a guide to different types of restaurants, but one that takes healthy eating options into consideration. If you're an afternoon in-the-office snacker, you could plan in advance and bring a healthy snack to work, like some fruit.

The National Weight Control Registry (NWCR) has a roster of approximately five thousand people and counting who have lost thirty pounds or more and have kept off this weight for at least a year. Their findings show that the main reason people have kept off the weight is—no surprise here—exercise. Ninety-four percent increased their physical activity, and the most popular activity is walking. But the second reason might surprise you: *98 percent* of NWCR participants modified the way they ate. Another way to think about that statistic is that 98 percent of these weight-loss success stories involved taking some basic dieting ideas and making them their own.[3] This means being proactive rather than passively eating what a "parent" diet tells you is okay. It means treating yourself like an adult who can make his or her own decisions and discover ways to modify your eating in order to maintain weight loss.

It takes a certain amount of creative thinking. And to jump-start this way of thinking, I am now going to give you a list of some creative tips that I've given my clients to help them lose weight—and keep it off. Remember, this isn't a diet, and some of these tips may be right for you and some not.

Some Creative Tips to Help You Lose Weight for Life

- **Give almond butter a try.** It's a healthier snack than peanut butter—almonds are rich in protein and the fat they contain is a healthy kind of fat—and it tastes delicious! Try it on a piece of spelt bread, a fiber-rich grain with fewer calories than regular bread.
- **Freeze grapes or bananas** and munch on them for snacks.
- **Use plain nonfat yogurt instead of sour cream** on a baked potato (or, as I prefer, on a boiled cassava).
- **Eat a handful of raw almonds before a big event.** It'll keep you satiated and less tempted by the buffet.
- **Or if almonds aren't your thing, try other nuts, beans, lentils, or fish.** All are great sources of lean protein.
- **Order salad dressing on the side**, then use your fork to add the minimum amount to make your salad taste good.
- **Don't eat anything that is incapable of rotting.** This is just a good rule of thumb—"live foods" tend to contain the most healthy kinds of fats and oils, and don't contain all the harmful preservatives.
- **Eat before you are famished.** If you wait until you're virtually starving to eat, you will almost certainly end up overeating.
- **Precut and preprepare your snacks and your meals.** By doing so, you will have the opportunity to think in advance about the kinds of foods you're eating—and less likely to grab something unhealthy on the spur of the moment.
- **Put individual portions of cereal, oatmeal, or pasta in containers or plastic bags.** You'll be less tempted to reach for more.
- **Don't eat right before you go to bed.** The calories (fuel) you eat before you fall asleep won't get a chance to burn off and these calories are usually stored as fat.

- **Shop the outside aisles of your supermarket.** The processed, fatty, and fake foods are usually kept in the middle aisles.
- **Don't go food shopping when you are hungry!** It's just too tempting.
- **Keep raw veggies handy.** Baby carrots, celery, string beans, jicama—these will fill you up without filling you out.
- **Look for the words "grilled," "poached," and "roasted" on a menu.** These will help ensure you're not going to get a lot of heavy, calorie-laden foods.
- **Stay away from "creamy" foods.** Sauces, soups, and salad dressing made with cream are much more fattening—and more dangerous to your heart—than their vinaigrette, tomato, or broth-based counterparts.
- **Say no to fried foods.** Your heart will thank you! Deep-fried foods not only mean extra calories but also a lot of additional saturated and trans fats, which are bad for your cholesterol and can cause heart disease.
- **Don't buy foods that tempt you.** In other words, keep cookies, chips, and ice cream out of the house. Enjoy your treats when you are out only.
- **Invest in a grill.** Grilling is one of the ultimate high-flavor, low-fat cooking methods, because a lot of the fat can be cooked away from the food. It's also a great way to flash-heat vegetables for a sweeter taste.
- **Eat egg whites instead of whole eggs.** They have fewer calories and are healthier for your heart.
- **Use real fruit jams.** They taste delicious and have far fewer calories and preservatives than traditional jams.
- **Stay away from sugar-free.** It seems counterintuitive, but if you check out the ingredients on a sugar-free cookie or jam, you'll find a lot more fat, a lot more artificial ingredients, and, most of the time, exactly the same calories!
- **Avoid high-fructose corn syrup.** High-fructose corn syrup (HFCS) is found in almost everything we eat today. Food manufacturers love it because of its low cost and long shelf life. Unlike other carbohydrates, HFCS does not cause the pancreas to produce insulin, which acts as a hunger-quenching signal to the brain, so you just keep eating. Also, foods with HFCS are usually high in calories and low in nutritional value—which is reason alone to stay away from HFCS.
- **Limit the amount of diet soda you drink.** Yes, you know it's unhealthy. But did you know it can stimulate your appetite, too? A study found

that 41 percent of people who drink diet soda are more likely to be obese.[20] If you crave the sparkle, try drinking seltzer with a drop of pomegranate juice or lemon and lime.

■ **Wipe out white.** White rice, white sugar, white flour pasta, white bread . . . replace these do-nothing carbs with whole-grain breads, whole-grain pastas, brown rice, and organic brown sugar, agave, or honey!

■ **Eat breakfast.** I especially recommend starting your day with whole-grain cereal or oatmeal. People who eat breakfast are almost half as likely to suffer from heart disease, diabetes, or obesity.[23] Fiber-rich whole-grain cereal will fill you up faster, so you'll eat less throughout the day[24]

■ **Multivitamin supplements.** If you want assurance that you're getting all the vitamins and minerals your body needs, a multivitamin is a great complement to a healthy balanced diet. (Always talk to your doctor about which supplements might be right for you.)

POWERtips >> RAISING THE BAR. Nutritional bars make excellent snacks, but some are more nutritious than others. I prefer raw, organic, cold-processed bars. Why? Because raw, living foods are clean and have a higher nutrient content than cooked food. Raw organic bars are alkaline-forming, which provides your body an environment that is healing and healthy—for both ourselves and global ecology.

The nutrition bars I recommend are:
Lara Bar: *www.larabar.com*
Raw Indulgence: *www.rawindulgence.com*
The Pure Bar: *www.thepurebar.com*
The Organic Food Bar: *www.organicfoodbar.com/products*
Greens+ Chocolate Energy Bar: *www.greensplus.com*

So now you have an idea of how to make your diet your own. But what about the food itself? How can you guarantee you're eating a well-balanced, healthy diet?

CALORIES, CARBS, PROTEINS, FATS, AND JUICING

When it comes to maintaining a healthy diet and losing excess weight, there are five main things to keep in mind: calories, carbs, proteins, fats, and juicing. You probably hear these words a lot, but there's a lot of mystery surrounding them, so it's important that we understand exactly what we're talking about. Let's go over each one:

Calories

Calories are measurements of energy. It's simple math: **3,500 calories equals one pound of fat.**

So burning 3,500 calories means losing one pound of fat. There's a very basic equation when it comes to weight loss and it is:

Burn more calories than you consume.

Men 19–50 should consume between 2,200 and 2,600 calories per day. Women 19–50 should consume between 1,800 and 2,200 calories per day. If you are active, you will burn more calories. Your metabolism stays high, your energy stays strong, and you do less emotional and unconscious eating. In fact, the more active you are, the better food choices you will *want* to make. The one thing leads to the other. It feels good to be active, and it inspires you to want to *extend* that good feeling with healthy eating habits.

Carbs

Carbs are the most common source of energy found in food.

Refined might be good when it comes to manners, but not when it comes to your health. Refined grains are stripped of all their nutrients, and when you add refined sugar and fat (the three are usually found together) you have an artery just waiting to be clogged.

But carbs themselves have gotten a bad rep. Not all carbs are bad. Whole grains are vital for a nutrition-rich diet because they are rich in fiber and a great source of energy. Refined grains break down quickly and make the liver work hard churning out insulin for energy—a danger for those at risk for diabetes. Whole grains take much longer to break down due to the fiber and, therefore, require less insulin production and provide energy for sustained periods of time. Good carbs are unprocessed carbohydrates in their natural state; pretty much all leafy vegetables and fruits fit into this category.

And the best incentive to choose whole grains when you're trying to lose weight? High fiber makes you feel fuller with fewer calories. It has also been found to help reduce bad cholesterol in the blood.[5]

POWERtips >> **GHRELIN AND LEPTIN.** These two words might sound like a mouthful, but they are also very intimately *involved* in a mouthful. Both are hormones that affect our feelings of satiety and hunger. Leptin suppresses our appetite. Produced in your fat cells, it signals you to stop eating when those cells are full.

Ghrelin is the evil twin of leptin; it has the opposite effect. It stimulates appetite. The more ghrelin in your system, the more hungry you become and the more you eat—and store fat.

Whenever we reduce our food intake to lose weight, ghrelin is stimulated. The more restrictive the diet, the more ghrelin is stimulated and the hungrier you become. What happens next? A food binge. That's what happens when we can't stand it anymore. We binge—which produces leptin and makes us feel full. It is this relationship that makes long-term dieting success difficult. You can't restrict your calories to the point of starvation without your body—that wonderful, finely tuned machine—acting up. In fact, the more low-fat the diet, the worse it gets. This is part of the reason why low-fat or no-fat diets don't work. Fat helps stimulate more leptin and keeps you full. Without any fat, you're going to be twice as hungry (not to mention the dry skin and lack of energy). But that doesn't mean loading up on the Twinkies. We're talking healthy fats here: nuts, fish oils, olive oils, and avocados.

The ghrelin-leptin phenomenon is the reason I tell my clients to eat a handful of raw almonds before an event or party. The fat helps stimulate leptin fast—which will make you less hungry. A bonus? They taste good and do good things for your body.[6,7]

Protein

Protein is a long chain of amino acids linked together. Also known as the building block of life, protein's most important function is to build, maintain, and replace tissue in our bodies. Our muscles, organs, and some of our hormones are made up of mostly protein. Proteins are involved in almost every function performed by a cell. Without protein, life would be impossible. Our body is able to produce only some of the amino acids (protein) we need. The remaining (known as essential amino acids) must be obtained through our diets. Great protein sources include fish, avocados, beans, soy, dairy, nuts, and white-meat poultry.

But if I asked you what kinds of foods contain protein (or more specifically, these essential amino acids), your first answer would probably be meat. The problem, however, is that meat—and while we're at it, all animal products—contain cholesterol. So if you're looking for a healthier alternative, something with heart-health benefits and none of the risk associated with meat, you should try plant-source proteins instead. We now have clear evidence that a diet derived exclusively from the vegetable kingdom can provide all the essential amino acids for optimal health.

Some proof:

- In three weeks on a plant-based diet, overweight subjects lost, on average, seventeen pounds.[8]
- At the Pritikin Center, people who ate a plant-based, low-fat healthy diet lost approximately 5.5 percent of their body weight in three weeks.[9]
- Another study found their subjects lost approximately ten pounds in three weeks.[10]
- People who have the most weight to lose are the ones who lose the most weight when they start a low-fat, plant-based diet.[11]

I understand some people love their meat and don't want to give it up. That's okay, but you should stick to organic, free-range, grass-fed sources—and try the healthier options, like lean beef. Also, give white-meat poultry a try, or fish and seafood. You might like it more than you think!

Fats

Most foods contain some type of fat and some are better for you than others. Fat is a necessary nutrient. Our bodies need it in order to function properly. It helps in our energy production and our blood clotting; it helps to regulate blood pressure and to maintain a healthy nervous system; it carries fat-soluble vitamins from your food in the body; and your skin, hair, and nails all depend on it.

But eating the wrong kinds of fat can be harmful and can lead to weight gain, diabetes, heart disease, and cancer.

Let me break it down for you.

There are **healthy, good fats,** and they include the following:

- monounsaturated fat: olives, avocados, nuts
- polyunsaturated fat: vegetable oils, cereals, bananas, hemp seeds
- omega-3 fatty acids: fish, flax, walnuts

Then there are **unhealthy, bad fats**, and they include:

- saturated fat: animal products such as meat, dairy and eggs, also found in some plant-based sources such as coconut and palm oils
- trans fat: hydrogenated oils found in cookies, crackers, cakes, and also common in fried foods, like donuts and french fries
- cholesterol: animal products, dairy, organs

Being aware of the kinds of fats you eat, and trying to stick to the good, healthy ones, is crucial to your health.

Juicing

Most of us don't get the vegetables we need on a daily basis. The National Cancer Society and the U.S. Department of Agriculture recommend at least five servings of vegetables and four of fruit a day—but the average American eats only one and a half servings of vegetables a day and zero fruit![21]

How to fit in your five servings a day? In a word: juicing.

If you buy only one item after reading this book, make it a juicer. It is an investment for your health—today and in the future. Not only will a daily juice give you the vegetables your body craves, but also chlorophyll, a plant-based substance that may help your blood transport life-sustaining oxygen to your system, and enzymes that strengthen and aid your digestive tract, metabolic activity, and cellular food absorption.

Even better news: Juicers are more convenient than ever, with easy-to-clean containers. You don't need a cookbook to make juice. Be creative. Try a mix of different types of fruits and vegetable, as much and as many as you want.

Here are some of the fruits and vegetables that I juice and recommend:

1. **Celery.** A vegetable with high calcium content, it's also an excellent diuretic that's good for the kidneys. It helps in the elimination of body waste through the urine.

2. **Carrots.** This hearty cancer fighter is rich in beta-carotene and many essential vitamins and minerals.

3. **Cucumbers.** Where do I start? This vegetable is high in silica, a mineral that strengthens connective tissue—which makes it beneficial for tendons, muscles, cartilage, bones, and ligaments. Studies show that silica is also good for maintaining your skin elasticity and smooth complexion, keeping fingernails strong, and preventing hair loss. *But please note: Use organic or nonwaxed cucumbers, which don't need peeling because most of the silica and other vitamins and minerals are in its skin.*

4. **Spinach.** This health booster aids our digestive process. Organic, raw spinach cleans our intestines and improves their function. Two cups (or half a liter) of fresh spinach juice every day can help get rid of the worst bouts of constipation within days or weeks.

5. **Ginger.** Not only will this add a spicy "tang" to your juice, but because of its protein-digesting power, ginger will stimulate the bile that digests fat, as well as promote the growth of healthy intestinal flora. It not only helps restore proper digestive function, but it also contains many antioxidants.

6. **Lemon.** A small fruit with a mighty wallop, lemon helps prevent and treat many ailments, including liver problems, gallstones, infection, high fever, asthma, urinary tract infections, arthritis, and sore throat.[22]

7. **Parsley.** It's not just a garnish anymore. **Parsley contains three times as much vitamin C as oranges and twice as much iron as spinach!** It's also an excellent source of vitamins A and K, folate, and more.

8. **Garlic** contains allicin, an antibiotic compound that has been used for centuries to fight infection.

9. **Beets** are to juices as apple is to core (which is also an excellent sweetener for a juice). Beets are rich in natural sugar and contain sodium, potassium, phosphorus, calcium, sulfur, chlorine, iodine, iron, copper, vitamins B_1, B_2, C, and P (bio flavonoids)—all of which help clean the kidneys and gallbladder. Beets are easily digestible carbohydrates with a low caloric content.

POWERFUL SUPERFOODS

There are healthy foods, and then there are *uber*-healthy foods, or what I think of as "superfoods." If you try to eat one or more of the following superfoods—all readily available and convenient to use—every day, your power will soar!

Superfood #1: Almonds

Power Eating: Raw with skins intact
Superpowers: Building muscles and fighting food cravings
Secret Weapons: Protein, monounsaturated fats, vitamin E, folate, fiber, magnesium, phosphorus
Fighting Against: Obesity, heart disease, muscle loss, cancer
Superpower Sidekicks: Pumpkin seeds, sunflower seeds
Impostors: Salted or smoked nuts. High sodium spikes blood pressure!

Superfood #2: Beans

Power Eating: Soak raw until soft, then cook
Superpowers: Building muscles, helping to burn fat, regulating digestion
Secret Weapons: Fiber, protein, iron, folate
Fighting Against: Obesity, colon cancer, heart disease, high blood pressure
Superpower Sidekicks: Lentils, peas, bean dips, hummus, edamame
Impostors: Refried beans (high in saturated fat), baked beans (high in sugar)

Superfood #3: Spinach

Power Eating: Raw, steamed, juiced, or slightly sautéed
Superpowers: Neutralizing free radicals, the molecules that accelerate the aging process
Secret Weapons: Vitamins A, C, and K, folate, beta-carotene, minerals including calcium and magnesium, fiber
Fighting Against: Cancer, heat disease, stroke, obesity, osteoporosis
Superpower Sidekicks: Cruciferous vegetables, such as broccoli and Brussels sprouts; green, yellow, red, and orange vegetables, such as asparagus, peppers, and yellow beans
Impostors: None—as long as you don't fry them or smother them in fatty cheese sauces!

Superfood #4: Instant Oatmeal

Power Eating: Unsweetened and unflavored
Superpowers: Boosting energy and sex drive, reducing cholesterol, maintaining blood sugar levels
Secret Weapons: Complex carbohydrates, fiber
Fighting Against: Heart disease, diabetes, colon cancer, obesity
Superpower Sidekicks: High-fiber cereals, such as All-Bran and Fiber One
Impostors: Sugary cereals that claim to contain oats

Superfood #5: Olive Oil

Power Eating: Organic, extra-virgin
Superpowers: Lowering cholesterol, boosting the immune system, controlling food cravings, helping to burn fat

Secret Weapons: Monounsaturated fat (lowers bad cholestrol), vitamin E
Fighting Against: Obesity, cancer, heart disease, high blood pressure
Superpower Sidekicks: Canola, peanut, and sesame oils
Impostors: Other vegetable and hydrogenated vegetable oils, trans-fatty acids, margarine

Superfood #6: Almond Butter

Power Eating: On spelt or other whole-grain bread or cracker
Superpowers: Boosting testosterone, building muscle, helping to burn fat
Secret Weapons: Protein, monounsaturated fat, vitamin E, niacin, magnesium
Fighting Against: Obesity, muscle loss, wrinkles, cardiovascular disease
Superpower Sidekicks: Cashew and peanut butters
Impostors: Mass-produced sugary and trans-fatty peanut butters

POWERtips >> **Fiber-licious.** Soluble fiber forms a gel-like material in the intestines that prevents cholesterol and saturated fats from entering the bloodstream; it also plays a role in metabolizing blood sugar.

Insoluble fiber attracts water in your intestines, which helps increase bulk and ultimately soften stools and move carcinogens more quickly through your intestines in the form of excrement. Insoluble fiber will also keep you "regular."

Both types of fiber may prevent colorectal cancer. Soluble fiber is found in oat bran, nuts, flaxseed, oranges, apples, carrots, dried beans, and peas. Insoluble fiber is found in vegetables, fruit skins, root vegetable skins, wheat oat, seeds, and nuts.

Superfood #7: Blueberries

Power Eating: Raw or fresh frozen
Superpowers: Protecting the body from stress of day-to-day living, strengthening immune system, enhancing brain function
Secret Weapons: Anthocyanin, a superpowerful antioxidant with triple the stress-fighting power of vitamin C, and other antioxidants, vitamins, fiber
Fighting Against: Built-up stress, aging, cancer, memory loss, heart disease, urinary infection
Superpower Sidekicks: Strawberries, raspberries, blackberries

Impostors: Dried berries (although high in nutrients, also high in concentrated [sugar] calories)

Superfood #8: Oranges

Power Eating: Peeled and raw
Superpowers: Lowering cholesterol, inhibiting blood-clot formation, boosting immune system, maintaining blood-sugar levels, cancer
Secret Weapons: Vitamin C, flavonoids (phytonutrients that boost its superpowers), limonene (oil found in the peel that may inhibit certain cancers; grating peel brings an explosion of limonene scent)
Fighting Against: High cholesterol, stroke, myocardial infarctions, peripheral artery disease (PAD), high blood sugar, obesity, cancer
Superpower Sidekicks: Lemon, grapefruit, Ugli fruit
Impostors: Canned fruit with added sugar, mass-produced juice with preservatives

Superfood #9: Avocado

Power Eating: Raw, scooped out from peel
Superpowers: Neutralizing heart-disease risks, building muscles, fighting food cravings
Secret Weapons: Fiber, contains all essential amino acids and then some, unsaturated fat, vitamins C and B_6, folate
Fighting Against: Formation of homocysteine, a substance that may cause heart attacks, obesity, muscle loss, cancer
Superpower Sidekicks: Nuts and nut butters
Impostors: Guacamole (delicious, yes, but contains a high quantity of fat)

Superfood #10: Whole-Grain Cereals

Power Eating: With rice, almond, or soy milk in the morning
Superpowers: Suppressing appetite, helping to prevent heart disease, stabilizing blood sugar
Secret Weapons: Fiber, vitamins C and B_6, iron, folic acid, phytochemicals
Fighting Against: Colon cancer and other cancers, high cholesterol, obesity, diabetes

Superpower Sidekicks: Whole-grain organic breads and crackers
Impostors: Sugary cereals

Superfood #11: Tomatoes

Power Eating: Raw
Superpowers: Helping to prevent prostate, colon, and other cancers, promoting pancreatic health, reducing heart disease risk, improving cholesterol, reducing formation of blood clots
Secret Weapons: Lycopene, a powerful antioxidant, vitamins A and C, iron, carotenoids
Fighting Against: Heart disease, cancer, infection, stroke
Superpower Sidekicks: Other vegetables and fruit
Impostors: Mass-produced pasta and pizza sauces

POWERtips >> QUINOA IS ONE of the single most complete food sources on Earth. It is rich in protein and it is one of the only grains that contain all of the essential amino acids. As such it is a perfectly balanced food and a great substitute for animal products. Also it's rich in calcium, high in iron, phosphorus, E and several B vitamins. And it's wheat- and gluten-free. I eat it cold in salads with beans and vegetables, hot in place of rice, and also in wraps with hummus and avocado and tomato. There are so many ways to prepare it that with a little creativity you'll find yourself enjoying this perfect food all the time.

Superfood #12: Quinoa

Power Eating: Unsweetened, cooked as cereal
Superpowers: Promoting a balanced diet all by itself
Secret Weapons: Carbohydrates, protein (contains all essential amino acids), good fat, fiber, calcium, iron, potassium, folic acid, magnesium, vitamin B_6, zinc
Fighting Against: Cancer, heart disease, vitamin and mineral deficiencies, weakness, infection
Superpower Sidekicks: None; quinoa is one of the single most complete food sources.

Impostors: Other grains (although good for you, most other grains aren't as complete and balanced a food)

Superfood #13: Milled Flaxseeds

Power Eating: Sprinkled on salad, over oatmeal, cooking
Superpowers: Strengthening the immune system, helping to protect against cancer, diabetes, and heart disease, strengthening bone-density mass (BDM)
Secret Weapons: Fiber, omega-3 fatty acids, antioxidants, vitamin B, magnesium
Fighting Against: Autoimmune disease, heart disease, diabetes, cancer, osteoporosis
Superpower Sidekicks: Wheat germ, bran
Impostors: None, but flaxseeds can get rancid quickly; store in refrigerator. And be sure to buy milled; our bodies don't digest whole flaxseeds.

Superfood #14: Green Tea

Power Eating: Hot or cold.
Superpowers: Improving immune function, lowering LDL cholesterol levels
Secret Weapons: Epigallocatechin gallate (EGCG), a powerful antioxidant, which inhibits the growth of cancer cells and kills existing cancer cells without harming healthy tissue
Fighting Against: Cancer, rheumatoid arthritis, high cholesterol, CVD (cardiovascular disease)
Superpower Sidekicks: None
Impostors: Sugary drinks with green tea in them

Superfood #15: Cranberries

Power Eating: Juiced
Superpowers: Fighting infection, improves circulatory system.
Secret Weapons: Antioxidants, rich in vitamin C, anti-inflammatory effects
Fighting Against: urinary infections, plaque on teeth, stomach ulcers, tumors
Superpower Sidekicks: None
Impostors: Dried cranberries

Superfood #16: Pineapple

Power Eating: Peeled and raw or juiced
Superpowers: Boosting the immune system, helping maintain good eye health, anti-inflammatory
Secret Weapons: Calcium, potassium, fiber, and vitamin C (antioxidants), bromelain (anti-inflammatory), manganese
Fighting Against: Arthritis, gum disease, heart disease
Superpower Sidekicks: None
Impostors: Canned pineapple with added sugar

Superfood #17: Mango

Power Eating: Peeled, raw
Superpowers: Aiding with digestion, known as blood builders because of their high iron content
Secret Weapons: Antioxidants, iron, vitamins A and E, selenium
Fighting Against: Heart disease, cervical cancer, colon cancer, anemia
Superpower Sidekicks: None
Impostors: None

Superfood #18: Turmeric

Power Eating: As a spice, also found in yellow mustard
Superpowers: Known as one of nature's most powerful healers in India (and used in almost all foods), where the incidence of our top four cancers (colon, breast, prostate, and lung) is said to be ten times lower
Secret Weapons: Antioxidant, anti-inflammatory
Fighting Against: Cancer, oxidative damage
Superpower Sidekicks: None
Impostors: Seasonings full of sodium-containing turmeric

Superfood #19: Pomegranates

Power Eating: Juiced
Superpowers: Antioxidant
Secret Weapons: Neutralize free radicals that cause disease

Fighting Against: Breast cancer, lung cancer, prostate cancer, Alzheimer's, high-LDL cholesterol, high blood pressure
Superpower Sidekicks: All berries
Impostors: Sugary juices

EATING ORGANIC!

Is eating organic that much better for you than eating conventional foods? In my opinion, YES!

Eating organic is not only good for us and our bodies but also for our planet. It's good for our health because eating organic reduces an individual toxin's burden of pesticides and food additives. But it's also good for Mother Earth because organic farmers use less energy, less water resources, and no pesticides or other harmful chemicals that pollute our environment.

Organic foods contain a greater amount of vitamins and minerals than inorganic foods because of the fast, cheap production and fertilizers that destroy many of the nutrients in inorganic foods.

But can I afford it? you ask. YES! Recent studies have shown that the average family spends more on junk food, takeaway, alcohol, and tobacco than on fruits and vegetables. So cut back on the stuff you don't need and load up on delicious, health-promoting organic foods!

MAKING YOUR EATING PROGRAM WORK FOR YOU

To give you a jump start on your healthy eating behavior, here are three sample menus. Each one includes a good healthy version of one of the elements we talked about above—calories, carbs, protein, fats, and juices—and each includes at least three superfoods. These menus are designed to be adaptable: You can use them at home, at work, or at a restaurant. You can also mix and match, exchanging one lunch or dinner with another.

I've added portion size only in those foods that may need a watchful eye in the beginning of your new healthy lifestyle, especially if you want to lose weight. The caloric content of each menu is approximately 1,200 to 1,800, depending on your portion size.

Add fruits and vegetables as snacks as necessary.

Menu #1:

Breakfast: 1 cup oatmeal w/rice or almond milk and an orange
Snack: Baby carrots
Lunch: Spinach salad (walnuts, tomatoes, cucumber, avocado, and chickpeas), with oil and vinegar on the side
Snacks: Handful of almonds
       Apple
Juice: Celery/beet/cucumber/carrot
Dinner: Grilled halibut
       1 cup brown rice with broccoli
Snack: Raspberries

Menu #2:

Breakfast: 1 slice whole-grain bread with almond butter and fresh blueberries
       Grapefruit
Snack: Pear
Lunch: Veggie burger on spelt bread with mustard
       Tossed salad with balsamic vinegar dressing on side
Snack: Sliced strawberries
Juice: Carrot/apple/parsley/zucchini
Dinner: Poached salmon with fresh dill, parsley, and pepper
       Steamed broccoli and spinach
       Baked yam
Snack: 1 cup dry oatmeal with sliced mango

Menu #3:

Breakfast: 1 cup hemp granola cereal with rice, almond, or soy milk, milled flax and blackberries
Snack: *Juiced* celery and apple (seeds removed before juicing)
Lunch: Mesclun salad with grilled salmon, walnuts, pine nuts, and sliced pineapple
       Homemade honey mustard dressing (organic yellow mustard mixed with balsamic vinegar)

Snack: Raw, organic nutrition bar

Juice: Lemon/beet/turnip/cucumber/ginger

Dinner: Black and red pinto beans seasoned with garlic and cumin
        1 cup quinoa

Snack: Apple with cashew butter

POWER EATING RECAP

Remember, this is a lifestyle program, not a diet. It's not a race.

Ease into Power Eating, jump right to the menu samples, or plan how you want to start and when. There's no right way. And more important, there is no wrong way.

Just remember the following and you'll do fine:

✓ **Be mindful of calories, carbs, protein, fats, and juicing:**
1. Consume fewer calories (and burn more with exercise).
2. Eat healthy proteins: more plant-based.
3. Choose whole-grain carbohydrates.
4. Choose healthy kinds of fats.
5. Juice, building up to once a day.

✓ **Adapt these good habits to your particular lifestyle:**
1. Answer the questions in this chapter and analyze your responses in order to pinpoint your style.
2. Follow tips that work *for you.*
3. Eat like you mean it—slowly and fully.

✓ **Be aware of diet mind traps:**
1. One bagel or burger does not mean you "blew" it.
2. Avoid emotional eating.
3. Never deprive yourself, just be aware of your goals and weigh the risk versus reward.

✓ **Remember: This is a journey, not a destination:**
Healthy eating is only a spoonful away. Every day is an opportunity to be a healthier, fitter, and better you.

Conclusion

"CONSISTENCY is key."

THE POWER MOVES TOP 10

The following is a short list of the top ten things I want you to take away from this book . . .

1. **Almost all of the important exercise we do "hinges" on these four joints:**
   - Shoulders
   - Elbows
   - Hips
   - Knees

   Exercising these four joints will help you on your way toward optimum health and a beautiful, powerful, healthy body.

2. **There are three basic Power Moves exercise programs.** These are made for a range of scenarios or fitness levels. You should start with the first one and move up to the third.
   - The No-Excuses Workout
   - The Maintain/Stay-in-the-Game Workout
   - The Warrior Workout

3. **Each workout can be adapted to any situation.** For example, if you normally do the Warrior workout but, say, you're traveling on business and have no equipment and/or limited time, then you can simply up the reps on the No-Excuses workout to get your Power Moves in.

4. **Do cardiovascular aerobic exercise at least three times a week.** Walking can be done anywhere, anytime, and is among the safest exercises you can do. Once you are familiar with your Power Moves workout, you can get

extra cardio in by jumping rope or running in place between moves. You can also do each move faster to keep your heart rate up.

5. **Warm up for up to fifteen minutes** before starting your Power Moves workout and *take five minutes to cool down* after your exercise regimen. And don't forget to stretch.

6. **Juice** once a day.

7. **Be mindful of what you eat . . .**
   - Whole grains
   - Lean protein
   - Good fats
   - Fruits and vegetables

8. **To lose weight, you need to burn more calories than you consume.** Remember this formula: 3,500 calories = 1 pound of fat.

9. **Eat at least one Superpower Food every day.** These foods are rich in antioxidants, vitamins, minerals, protein, and fiber. Your body will love you for it and you will love your body for it as well.

10. **Consistency is key. Keep your eye on the big picture to stay motivated, YOUR HEALTH!**

Appendix A

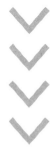

BODY FAT VERSUS LEAN MUSCLE

Although most people's primary motivation for weight loss is to improve their appearance, there are also many health benefits. And in order to stay lean and healthy, it is very important to know and understand your body-fat-to-muscle ratio. Excess body fat is linked to major health threats like heart disease, cancer, diabetes, and stroke—all of which are leading causes of death every year. Knowing your body fat stats also allows you to set realistic goals for weight loss.

The term "obese" specifically refers to an excessive amount of body fat. "Overweight" refers to an excessive amount of body weight. Both terms are used to describe an amount greater than what is considered healthy.

BODY MASS INDEX (BMI)

Body Mass Index is determined by a simple equation: a person's weight (in kilograms) divided by his or her height (in meters) squared. Generally a BMI of 25 or above is considered overweight and a value above 30 is considered obesity, which places the individual at an even higher risk of disease and health problems.

It is important to note that BMI has its limitations. BMI does not distinguish between fat and muscle or location of fat. Also, BMI is not a reliable indicator for most athletes, as well as many elderly or sickly individuals who have lost weight due to illness.

Many use BMI to classify fatness, and I believe caution must be used when doing so because BMI does *not* measure FAT. Two people may have very different body fat percentages and have the same BMI.

To use the table, find the appropriate height in the left-hand column labeled "Height." Move across to a given weight (in pounds). The number at the top of the column is the BMI at that height and weight. Pounds have been rounded off.

BMI Height (inches)	19	20	21	22	23	24	25	26	27	28	29	30	31	32	33	34	35
	Body Weight (pounds)																
58	91	96	100	105	110	115	119	124	129	134	138	143	148	153	158	162	167
59	94	99	104	109	114	119	124	128	133	138	143	148	153	158	163	168	173
60	97	102	107	112	118	123	128	133	138	143	148	153	158	163	168	174	179
61	100	106	111	116	122	127	132	137	143	148	153	158	164	169	174	180	185
62	104	109	115	120	126	131	136	142	147	153	158	164	169	175	180	186	191
63	107	113	118	124	130	135	141	146	152	158	163	169	175	180	186	191	197
64	110	116	122	128	134	140	145	151	157	163	169	174	180	186	192	197	204
65	114	120	126	132	138	144	150	156	162	168	174	180	186	192	198	204	210
66	118	124	130	136	142	148	155	161	167	173	179	186	192	198	204	210	216
67	121	127	134	140	146	153	159	166	172	178	185	191	198	204	211	217	223
68	125	131	138	144	151	158	164	171	177	184	190	197	203	210	216	223	230
69	128	135	142	149	155	162	169	176	182	189	196	203	209	216	223	230	236
70	132	139	146	153	160	167	174	181	188	195	202	209	216	222	229	236	243
71	136	143	150	157	165	172	179	186	193	200	208	215	222	229	236	243	250
72	140	147	154	162	169	177	184	191	199	206	213	221	228	235	242	250	258
73	144	151	159	166	174	182	189	197	204	212	219	227	235	242	250	257	265
74	148	155	163	171	179	186	194	202	210	218	225	233	241	249	256	264	272
75	152	160	168	176	184	192	200	208	216	224	232	240	248	256	264	272	279
76	156	164	172	180	189	197	205	213	221	230	238	246	254	263	271	279	287

Source: National Institutes of Health

Here's what the numbers mean:

If your BMI is:	You are considered:
Below 18.5	underweight
18.5–24.9	normal
25.0–29.9	overweight
30.0 and above	obese

ABDOMINAL FAT

Abdominal fat is considered by many health professionals to be the most danger-ous type of fat.

Abdominal fat is an important, independent risk factor for disease. Research has shown that waist circumference is directly associated with abdominal fat, which is called visceral or intra-abdominal fat. This type of fat is being linked to high cholesterol, elevated insulin levels, high blood pressure, and other health problems. If you carry fat mainly around your waist, you are more likely to devel-op obesity-related health problems.

Some experts say they don't know the optimal waist size for good health, while others share the opinion that women with a waist measurement of more than thirty-five inches and men with a waist measurement of more than forty inches may have more health risks than people with lower waist measurements because of their body fat distribution.

Whatever the case may be, it is clear that knowing your waist circumference is extremely important for maintaining optimum health.

BODY FAT PERCENTAGE

Hydrostatic weighing (underwater weighing) is the gold standard for calculating body fat. But although it is the most accurate, it's probably the least cost-effective. It's also quite inconvenient because it's time-consuming and not many places offer it.

"Fat calipers" are a great alternative. This is a low-cost, easy-to-use, portable option, and with some kinds of calipers you can even test yourself. Fat calipers measure skin folds to calculate how much subcutaneous fat (fat under the skin) a person has. These numbers are put into an equation that calculates body fat percentage. Although none of these methods is error-proof, fat calipers remain the favorite among many health professionals.

Appendix B
Helpful Resources

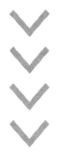

If you'd like additional information, here are some resources that I've found invaluable in my search for better health and fitness and some others that you may find fun and exciting . . .

Active.com
www.active.com

American Academy of Family
Physicians
www.familydoctor.org

American Heart Association
www.americanheart.org

Bikes To Go
www.bikestogo.com

Centers for Disease Control
www.cdc.gov

Duke Diet Center
www.dukedietcenter.org

Electra Bikes
www.eclectrabikes.com

GoVeg.com
www.goveg.com

Greens+
www.greensplus.com

Gym Source
www.gymsource.com

Happy Cow
www.happycow.net

Harvard School of Public Health
www.hsph.harvard.edu/nutritionsource

The Institute for Healthy Aging
www.antiagemed.com

iTunes
www.itunes.com

Kids Health
www.kidshealth.org

Lara Bar
www.larabar.com

Life Extension Foundation
www.lef.org

Living and Raw Foods
www.living-foods.com

Mayo Clinic
www/mayoclinic.com

Medline Plus
www.nlm.nih.gov/medlineplus/

National Institutes of Health
www.nih.gov

Organic.org
www.organic.org

Organic Food Bar
www.organicfoodbar.com/products

Personal Best/Oz Garcia
www.ozgarcia.com

Pritikin Longevity Center
www.pritikin.com

The Pure Bar
www.thepurebar.com

Raw Indulgence
www.rawindulgence.com

Real Age
www.realage.com

Whole Foods
www.wholefoodsmarket.com

Yoga Journal
www.yogajournal.com

Appendix C
Endnotes

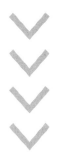

[1] Tuomilehto, J., Lindstrom, J., Eriksson, J. G., et al. "Prevention of type 2 diabetes mellitus by changes in lifestyle among subjects with impaired glucose tolerance." *New Engl J Med,* 2001, 344:1343–1350.

[2] Ornish, D. Brown, S. E., Scherwitz, L.W., et al. "Can lifestyle changes reverse coronary heart disease?" *Lancet,* 1990, 336:129–133.

[3] Campbell, T. C., Cambpell T. M. *The China Study: Startling Implications for Diet, Weight Loss and Long-Term Health.* Dallas, TX: BenBella Books, Inc., 2006, pp. 84–87.

[4] "Indoor cycling." Health A to Z. Available at www.healthatoz.com/healthatoz/Atoz/common/standard/transform.jsp?requestURI=/healthatoz/Atoz/hl/fit/card/spinning.jsp; accessed March 18, 2008.

[5] Gresl, T. A., Colman, R. J., Havighurst, T. C., et al. "Dietary restriction and b-cell sensitivity to glucose in adult male rhesus monkeys." *J Gerontol: Biological Sci,* 2003, 58A:45–57.

[6] University of Virginia. "Obesity in America." Available at www.healthsystem.virginia.edu/internet/occupational-health/obesityinamerica.pdf; accessed April 25, 2008.

[7] Nieman, P. "Childhood obesity." Available at www.dltk-kids.com/articles/childhood_obesity.htm; accessed April 25, 2009.

[8] University of Virginia. "Obesity in America." Available at www.healthsystem.virginia.edu/internet/occupational-health/obesityinamerica.pdf; accessed April 25, 2008.

[9] "Overweight." National Center for Health Statistics. Centers for Disease Control. Available at www.cdc.gov/nchs/fastats/overwt.htm; accessed March 18, 2008.

[10] Holt, J., Warren, L., Wallace, R. "What behavioral interventions are safe and effective for treating obesity?" *J Fam Med,* 2006, 55:536–538.

[11] "Rolls, B. J. "The supersizing of America: portion size and the obesity epidemic." *Nutrition Today,* 2003, 38:42–53.

[12] Verplanken, B., Myrbakk, V., Rudi, E. "The measurement of habit," in *The Routines of Decision-Making.* Betsch, T. and Haberstroh, S. (eds). Mahwah, NJ: Lawrence Erlbaum Books, 2005, pp. 231–247.

[13] Belza, B., Warms, C. "Physical activity and exercise in women's health." *Nurs Clin North Am,* 2004, 39:181–193.

[14] Christakis, N. A., Fowler, J. H. "The spread of obesity in a large social network over 32 years." *New Eng J Med,* July 2007, 357:370–379.

[15] Giada, F., Biffi, A., Agostoni, P. "Exercise prescription for the prevention and treatment of cardio-vascular diseases: part 1." *J Cardiovasc Med,* 2008, 9:529–544.

[16] Evans, R. "Weight watchers." *Allure,* April 2008, pp. 252–255.

[17] "Emotional eating." Available at http://www.medicinenet.com/emotional_eating/article.htm; accessed April 27, 2008.

[18] Yunsheng, M., Bertone, E. R., Stanek, E. J. "Association between eating patterns and obesity in a free-living US adult population." *Am J Epidem,* 2003, 158:85–92.

[19] "Aerobic exercise: what 30 minutes a day can do." Available at www.mayoclinic.com/health/aerobic-exercise/EP00002; accessed April 27, 2008.

[20] "Regular, moderate-to-vigorous aerobic exercise significantly reduces markers of increased colon-cancer risk in men." Fred Hutchinson Cancer Research Center. Available at: www.fhcrc.org/about/ne/news/2006/09/12/aerobic_exercise.html?&&printfriendly=yes; accessed April 20, 2008.

[21] Leonhardt, D. "5 tips from 'mindless eating.'" *New York Times* online. Available at www.nytimes.com/2007/05/02/bysubess/02davidside.html; accessed May 10, 2008.

[22] The National Weight Control Registry. Available at www.nwcr.ws/; accessed May 10, 2008.

[23] "Inside the pyramid." Available at www.mypyramid.gov/pyramid; accessed May 4, 2007.

[24] Kalra, S. P., Ueno, N., Kalra, P. S. "Stimulation of appetite by ghrelin is regulated by leptin restraint: peripheral and central sites of action." *Am Soc for Nutri Sci J,* 2005, 135:1331–1335.

[25] Editorial. "The stomach speaks—ghrelin and weight regulation." *N Engl J Med,* 2002, 346:1662–1663.

[26] Shintani, T. T., Hughes, C. K., Beckham, S., et al. "Obesity and cardiovascular risk intervention through the ad libitum feeding of traditional Hawaiian diet." *Am J Clin Nutr,* 1991, 53:1647(S)–1651(S).

[27] Barnard, R. J. "Effects of life-style modification on serum lipids." *Arch Intern Med,* 1991, 151:1389–1394.

[28] Ornish, D., Scherwitz, L. W., Doody, R. S., et al. "Effects of stress management training and dietary changes in treating ischemic heart disease." *JAMA,* 1983, 249:54–59.

[29] Feskanich, D., Willett, W. C., Colditz, G. A. "Calcium, vitamin D, milk consumption, and hip fractures: a prospective study among postmenopausal women." *Am J Clin Nutr,* 2003, 77(2):504–511.

[30] Warensjo, E., Jansson, J. H., Berglund, L., et al. "Estimated intake of milk fat is negatively associated with cardiovascular risk factors and does not increase the risk of a first acute myocardial infarction." *Br J Nutr,* 2004, 91:635–642.

[31] Chan J. M., Stampfer M. J., Ma J, Gann P. H., Gaziano J. M., Giovannucci E. "Dairy products, calcium, and prostate cancer risk in the Physicians' Health Study." *Am J Clin Nutr,* 2001;74:549–554.

[32] Tseng, M., Breslow, R. A., Graubard, B. I., Ziegler, R. G. "Dairy, calcium and vitamin D intakes and prostate cancer risk in the National Health and Nutrition Examination Epidemiologic Follow-up Study cohort." *Am J Clin Nutr,* 2005, 81:1147–1154.

[33] Cramer, D. W., Greenberg, E. R., Titus-Ernstoff, L., et al. "A case-control study of galactose consumption and metabolism in relation to ovarian cancer." *Cancer Epidemiol Biomarkers Prev,* 2000, 9:95–101.

[34] Larsson, S. C., Bergkvist, L., Wolk, A. "Milk and lactose intakes and ovarian cancer risk in the Swedish Mammography Cohort." *Am J Clin Nutr,* 2004, 80:1353–1357.

[35] Kushi, L. H., Mink, P. J., Folsom, A. R., et al. "Prospective study of diet and ovarian cancer." *Am J Epidemiol,* 1999, 149:21–31.

[36] Bertron, P., Barnard, N. D., Mills, M. "Racial bias in federal nutrition policy, part I: the public health implications of variations in lactase persistence." *J Natl Med Assoc,* 1999, 91:151–157.

[37] Rauramaa, P., Halonen, S. B., Vaisanen, T. A., et al. "Effects of aerobic physical exercise on inflammation and atherosclerosis in men: the DNASCO study. A six-year randomized, controlled trial." *Annals of Int Med,* 2004, 140:1007–1014.

[38] "The Benefits of Juicing." Living and Raw Foods. Available at www.living-foods.com/articles/benefits.html; accessed May 11, 2008.

[39] "The Health Benefits of Lemons." A 2 Z of Health, Beauty, and Fitness. Available at health.learninginfo.org/health-benefits-lemons.htm; accessed May 11, 2008.

[40] National Institute on Aging. "Chapter 4: sample exercises—stretching exercises." Available at www.nia.nih.gov/HealthInformation/Publications/ExerciseGuide/chapter04c.htm; accessed June 8, 2008.

[41] ScienceDaily. "Maintaining aerobic fitness could delay biological aging by up to 12 years, study shows." Available at www.sciencedaily.com/releases/2008/04/080409205827.htm; accessed June 8, 2008.

[42] ScienceDaily. "Low-intensity exercise reduces fatigue syndromes by 65 percent, study finds." Available at www.sciencedaily.com/releases/2008/080228112008.htm; accessed June 8, 2008.

[43] American Council on Exercise. "Studies show exercise can improve your sex life." Available at www.acefitness.org/fitfacts/fitfacts_display.aspx?itemid=159; accessed June 8, 2008.

Appendix D
Workout Cheat Sheet

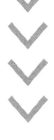

No-Excuses Workout

1. Squat Press

2. Reverse Lunge Press

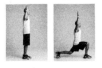

3. Single-Leg and Pelvic Lift

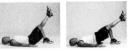

4. Push-Up into Side Plank

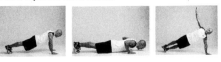

5. The Modified Cobra

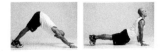

6. Reverse Dip

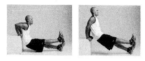

7. Pike Push-Up

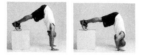

8. V-Ups

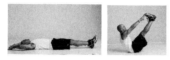

9. Modified Heel-Touch Crunch

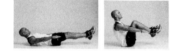

10. Straight-Leg Crunch

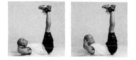

11. Upright Bicycle Crunch

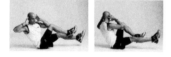

No-Excuses Resistance-Band Workout

1. Shoulder Fly Lunge

2. Reverse Chest Fly

3. Rows

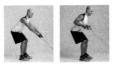

4. Biceps Curls

5. Triceps Kick

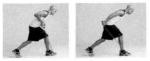

6. Shoulder Fly

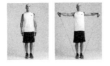

7. Reverse Crunch

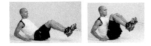

Maintain/Stay-in-the-Game Workout Option #1

1. Overhead Medicine Ball Squat

2. One-Arm Dumbbell Row

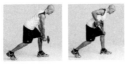

3. Medicine Ball Lunge and Twist

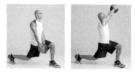

4. Incline Curl and Press

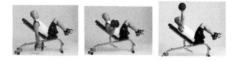

5. Bosu Ball Triceps Kick

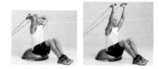

6. Medicine Ball Oblique Twist

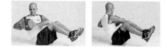

7. Resistance-Ball Jackknives

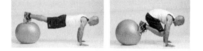

8. Medicine Ball Sit and Reach

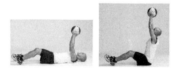

Maintain/Stay-in-the-Game Workout Option #2

1. Front and Back Lunge

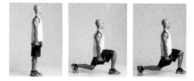

2. Horizontal Chin-Up

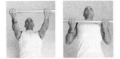

3. Spider Man Push-Up

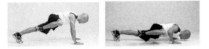

4. Good Morning Single-Leg Lift

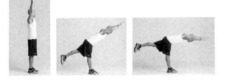

5. Burpies

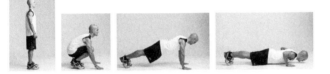

6. Plank

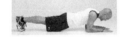

7. Medicine Ball Sit-Up Touch

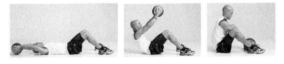

8. Resistance-Band Trunk Twist

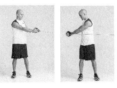

Maintain/Stay-in-the-Game Workout Option #3

1. Jumping Lunge

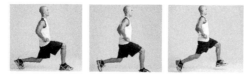

2. Hamstring Curl

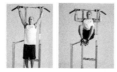

3. Pull-Up Blast

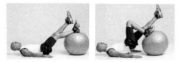

4. Resistance-Ball Chest Press

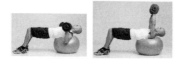

5. Reverse-Grip Barbell Curl

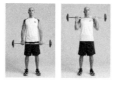

6. Overhead Dumbbell Extension

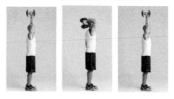

7. Dumbbell Shoulder Fly

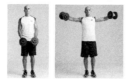

8. Oblique Side Plank

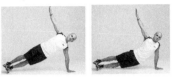

9. Medicine Ball Toe Touch

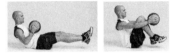

Warrior Workout Option #1

1. Deadlift High Pull

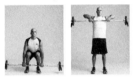

2. Single-Leg Dead Lift

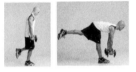

3. Romanian Split Squat

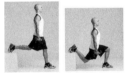

4. Bosu-Resistance Push-Up

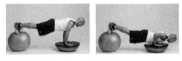

5. Towel Drag

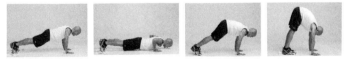

6. L Pull-Ups

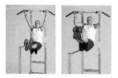

7. Single-Leg Dumbbell Curl

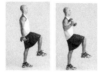

8. Parallel Dips

9. Suspended Resistance-Ball Sit-Up

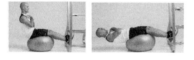

10. Forearm Planks

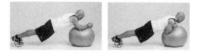

11. The Barbell Oblique Twist

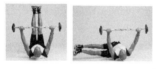

12. Figure 8s

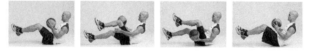

13. Single-Leg Plank

Warrior Workout Option #2

1. Dumbbell Front Squat

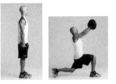

2. Reverse Lunge with Chest Fly

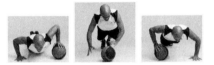

3. Exploding Push-Ups

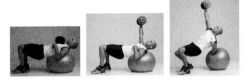

4. Resistance-Ball Single-Arm Press

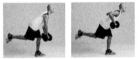

5. Single-Leg Dumbbell Row

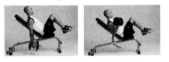

6. Incline Biceps Curls

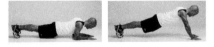

7. Triceps Plank Press

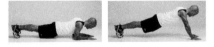

8. Dumbbell Shoulder Snatch

9. Hanging Knee Raises

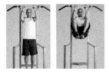

10. Reach and Touch

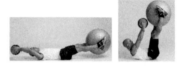

11. Plank Twist

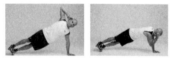

12. Incline Bench Reverse Crunch

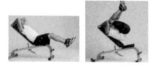

13. Resistance Chop

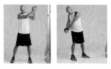

Try This!

1. Medicine Ball Pistol Squat

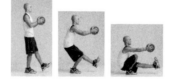

2. Dumbbell Jump-Through

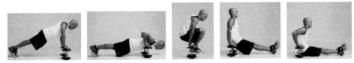

3. Barbell Oblique Toe Touch

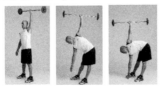

4. Medicine Ball Sit-Up & Stand

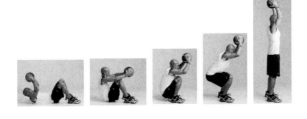

Power Stretching

1. Hamstring Stretch

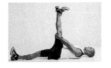

2. Kneeling Hip Flexor/Quad Stretch

3. Lying Trunk Twist

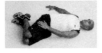

4. Overhead Lat Stretch

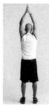

5. Chest Stretch

6. Standing Biceps Stretch

7. Triceps Overhead

8. Cross-Body Shoulder Stretch

Acknowledgments

This book would not have been possible without the help of many people:

Raymond Garcia, my brilliant publisher, thank you for your incredible vision and confidence in a project that started only as thoughts. When we met it was just for the purpose of this book, but in the process you've become a great friend.

Karla Dougherty, you brought this book to life, and for that I am eternally grateful.

Mark Chait, you have my utmost gratitude for your patience, keen sight, and ability to turn thoughts into crisp, clean words.

Jon Moe, thanks for giving extraordinary images to these motions. You're a gifted photographer and a great friend.

Eric Rovner, and the team at WMA, thanks to all of you for your support and faith.

My sister, Jennifer, thank you for pushing my abilities and for testing my determination.

My mother, Esther, and brother, Alfredo, if I never give up, it's because I learned it from you. Thank you.

My uncle Paul, the first person I actually saw lifting weights. He was the fittest man I knew, and it always inspired me. Thank you.

Last but not least, I would like to thank my wife, Marilyn, not only for giving me the greatest gift of my life, our son, but also for her love, endless support, and for not being afraid to dream with me.